Sleep, the Ultimate Bliss

There is nothing more beautiful than watching a baby sleeping. This same total surrender to sleep should be possible for all of us, throughout our lives.

But if you are currently suffering from that traumatic condition we call insomnia, I want to share with you the most effective techniques which we have developed over the last years for improving your night-time experience. No matter how hopeless you feel in the grip of insomnia, these realistic and gently powerful techniques can magically encourage the movement into peaceful sleep.

I write this book in the hope that you can take the suggestions and, without further help, advance into a new period of your life where sleep comes quickly and continues peacefully throughout each night!

John Selby

D1189593

SECRETS OF A GOOD NIGHT'S SLEEP

JOHN SELBY

AVON BOOKS ◢ NEW YORK

The techniques described in *Secrets of a Good Night's Sleep* have proven helpful for most insomniacs. However, in certain instances, the symptoms of insomnia reflect deeper problems. If, after working with the programs in this book, your symptoms persist, there may be an underlying medical cause which should be treated by a physician. Consult your doctor if you have any questions.

SECRETS OF A GOOD NIGHT'S SLEEP is an original publication of Avon Books. This work has never before appeared in book form.

AVON BOOKS
A division of
The Hearst Corporation
105 Madison Avenue
New York, New York 10016

Copyright © 1989 by John Selby
Published by arrangement with the author
Library of Congress Catalog Card Number: 89-91343
ISBN: 0-380-70815-9

First Avon Books Printing: December 1989

AVON TRADEMARK REG. U.S. PAT. OFF. AND IN OTHER COUNTRIES, MARCA REGISTRADA, HECHO EN U.S.A.

Printed in the U.S.A.

OPM 10 9 8 7 6 5 4 3 2 1

Contents

EASY-ACCESS INDEX TO SPECIAL SLEEP PROGRAMS

Foreword

People who are lucky enough not to suffer from insomnia have no idea how tortuous the condition can be. They can't even begin to imagine the trauma of being gripped by invisible inner tensions that simply refuse to let you relax and fall asleep night after night.

Recent statistics show that well over a quarter of the entire adult population in America suffer from one form or another of disrupted sleep patterns. This makes insomnia a major national health crisis, especially when one considers the immense economic and sociological impact of so many millions of people trying to get through a day following a series of sleepless nights.

What is the cause or multiple causes of insomnia, and more important, what can the average person do for him or herself to break free of insomnia's pernicious grip?

Traditionally, based on the medical approach to dealing with the problem, people suffering from sleeplessness have been treated mostly with sleeping pills and a few words of general life-style advice. Sleeping pills certainly do knock you out for a number of hours, but they do not induce natural sleep. Quite the opposite: they put your mind and body into a comatose state that bears little semblance to the various levels of activity of the sleeping mind.

Recently, scientific research has documented what doctors have been pointing out all along, that treating insomnia with drugs is not a cure for insomnia at all. Temporary relief might be induced, but in the long run sleeping pills create dependency and only treat surface symptoms, not the underlying causes of sleeplessness.

So where are we to turn for alternative ways of curing insomnia? First of all, new scientific studies have offered invaluable insights into the nature of insomnia. In this book I want to share with you the most important findings which shed light on why you can't fall asleep at night, and what you can realistically do to overcome your present condition.

Also, the wisdom and techniques of depth psychology and analysis, when combined with the recent scientific models,

1

offer important insights into a pragmatic approach to insomnia. I am a therapist myself and have worked with a number of my colleagues in developing effective programs for guiding clients beyond the maddening grip of sleeplessness. There also exist a number of special sleep clinics where intense therapy can be obtained.

But most people suffering from insomnia either cannot afford therapy, or simply don't feel their condition is so extreme as to justify lengthy professional help. Instead, they urgently need a practical and in-depth manual for helping themselves through the steps which have proven effective in inducing sleepful nights.

My intention in writing this book is to offer you in an easily accessible format the wisdom and pragmatic techniques which professionals work with in helping clients to overcome insomnia. My hope is that this book will become a non-drug "prescription" which doctors can recommend to their patients suffering from insomnia, so that there exists a realistic alternative to medication.

The inability to fall asleep at night is not a meaningless plague that grips us for no reason at all. There are very definite inner conditions which cause the symptom we call insomnia, and when our sleep becomes difficult and traumatic, it is extremely important to our overall well-being to pause and reflect on our present life situations, to discover the root provocation of our sleepless nights.

Sometimes people quickly get to the heart of their nocturnal restlessness, and learn to move into sleep quite easily. Other people need more time. You will find that you do have time to explore the programs offered in this book, because every night that you find yourself unable to sleep, you can open this book and continue with your inner reflections.

Curiously, your present problem of insomnia can quickly be transformed into a very worthwhile exploration, as you begin your journey to the headwaters of insomnia. Every new technique I offer you for inducing insight into your sleepless condition, and especially for inducing sleep itself, should prove quite enjoyable to explore and master moving you toward that most blissful of all experiences, the sleep you knew as a baby, the total surrender to your natural need for rest and recharging each night of your life.

I know personally in my own life, as well as in my work with clients, what it feels like to be caught tossing and turning in bed hour after hour, dreading the next day when you will be irritable and exhausted from too little sleep, but not knowing how to turn off your agitated thoughts and tensions that keep you away from sleep. There is a level of hopelessness and panic when you are caught in the grip of sleeplessness that is terrible to endure.

But no matter how hopeless you feel, I do want to say that help is at hand: there are realistic and gently powerful techniques you can learn readily in the pages to come that almost magically induce sleep. With each new chapter, I will take you further into mastering these techniques, so that by the time you have fully explored the entire book, you will know the primary professional, mental and emotional tools for successfully inducing sleep.

We will move forward on two fronts at the same time: learning steps you can immediately put to use to help you fall asleep this very night, and exploring the deeper reflections that will help you to understand and transcend the life situations that are generating your physical restlessness and mental agitation.

Along with the medical, psychological, and therapeutic approaches for overcoming insomnia, I have also drawn secular insights from the world's spiritual sources, such as the Christian contemplative and the Oriental meditation traditions, to offer basic help in attaining a deeper level of calm and peace in your life. Peace of mind is of course at the heart of a good night's sleep, so it is important to encourage this quality of consciousness, while also dealing with the more psychological techniques.

We spend a full third of our entire lives sleeping. It makes perfect sense to devote adequate time to understanding the sleep experience, to establish a more confident, positive relationship with our nightly journeys into the realms of sleep. I hope that this book offers you all the professional guidance and support you need for advancing into a bright new period of your life, where sleep comes quickly and continues peacefully throughout each night.

INTRODUCTION

Where Sleep Comes From

Quite a number of years ago I went with a guide into the Kalahari desert of southern Africa, where we stayed for a time with a small nomadic tribe of aborigines, living their life-style and getting to experience directly their ancient ways. Because one of my deepest insights into the nature of human sleep came to me during this adventure, I want to share the story with you.

There were only thirty members remaining of this tribe when I met them; essentially they were one big family, interacting now and then with other nomadic families in the region, but basically living their own tribal existence outside the confines of any civilization.

It was remarkable to my suburban eyes to get a glimpse into such an intimately knit extended family, where literally everyone interacted with everyone else in the family, every day, many times a day. There was a feeling of communal belonging which was quite total. Everything was owned in common, and sharing was the essence of all relating.

What I especially remember of this isolated tribal community was the feeling which came over the encampment when the sun headed for the western horizon of the desert and it came time to settle down for a night's sleep. The Kalahari is a somewhat dangerous place to sleep, out in the middle of nowhere, on the ground, with very real menaces walking around on padded cat's feet in the dead of night. But I seemed to be the only one who felt anxiety as darkness fell and left us sitting around a small fire.

One by one, first the children and old folks, then everyone else, would take their blanket and find a place to lie down to sleep. There didn't seem to be any special arrangements of who would sit up during what part of the night to watch out for danger, but it seemed that someone was always up tending the fire.

I felt acutely vulnerable and afraid, to be quite honest, as I got into my sleeping bag, and for the first couple of nights I could hardly sleep at all. But then I started to pick up on an amazing feeling in the night air, a feeling of not being alone, of belonging to this group of thirty people. I would watch the little children cuddling up beside their older sisters and brothers and parents. They were so trusting, as if the sum total of everyone's awareness in the tribe at night added up to more than enough watchfulness to protect them from harm.

And what I came to feel more and more as the days and nights went by was that there was a most remarkable quality of safety created by the communal living patterns of the small tribe. By staying intimately together, this family managed to survive, where alone each member would almost certainly perish in the desert.

And this feeling of communal participation seemed to generate an ability to fall asleep at night unafraid, even though the surroundings were somewhat dangerous. The more I tuned into this beautiful communal spirit, the easier I could sleep as well. I will never forget that special sensation of falling asleep while listening to thirty people breathing their way into sleep all around me. It was the ultimate family experience, and also an ultimate sleep experience.

I also remember with a shiver of fright how it felt to walk away from that wonderful desert family and to spend the following night alone with my guide in the vastness of the dark desert. I couldn't sleep a wink, it was so frightening to be sleeping alone without being surrounded by the aura of the family.

Then my guide and I returned to an encampment where

there were quite a few tourists staying, and that night was much better, sleeping in a real bed again, inside a house, safe from the elements. But still, I didn't sleep as well as I had out in the desert with the small tribe cuddled up on the ground together.

The important insight about the nature of sleep to be drawn from this experience is that human beings for countless generations have gathered together to sleep communally at night, both out of their desire to belong to a group and also out of necessity to gain protection. There is, without question, security in numbers.

Most of us were lucky enough to have had at least somewhat of a communal childhood; the very nature of the family, even the nuclear family, consists of at least a few people sleeping in close proximity. This primal feeling of communal security while sleeping is built into the very fabric of childhood family life. In fact, children in general have a very low incidence of insomnia, unless the basic family situation is disturbed. As long as Mom and Dad and perhaps some brothers and sisters are sleeping in the same house, there is a feeling similar to that which I felt so intensely among the tribe in the desert.

It has been found in sleep research that there are four levels to the sleep experience, as you have perhaps heard. We fall into a light sleep at first, from which we will awaken instantly if we hear a sound around us. Then we go into a somewhat deeper sleep for a few minutes. And then our brain waves show yet another shifting into a third level of sleep, where there comes a deeper relaxation, a quieting of thoughts and emotions.

And then, after about twenty minutes of sleeping time, we slip into an ultimate fourth state of total relaxation called delta sleep because of the unique brain-wave patterns at this level of sleeping. Such complete surrender to deep sleep is required by our minds and bodies each night if we are to awaken rested in the morning. But in this deep sleep, we are vulnerable to attack of any kind, since even loud noises will fail to awaken us.

If every member of the tribe in the Kalahari fell asleep into this deep delta sleep and stayed totally lost in sleep all through every night, the tribe would in fact be terribly vulnerable to attack. But here we find the essential fact about sleeping in communal situations which makes us able to relax at night.

After perhaps twenty minutes or so of delta sleep, we begin to rise upward through the different levels of sleep, toward consciousness again, or at least near-consciousness. Our minds become more active, we dream for a while, and during this near-waking state, any noises around us, any disturbances in the night, will wake us up. Then after half an hour or so, we again drift down into deep deep sleep for another cycle of complete relaxation and recharging.

If we are sleeping in a communal situation, some of us go to bed and fall asleep earlier than others, so there will always be some in the family who are down in delta sleep and completely gone to the world, while others are up to near-wakefulness, so that anything happening will cause full wakefulness and action.

Thus there is always someone on guard, so to speak. By the very nature of the sleep cycles in human beings, there is a built-in protection system in communal situations at night. And thus everyone can have time for complete delta sleep. A feeling of security is maintained, and insomnia avoided.

We repeat this basic cycle five times each night, as part of our genetic inheritance which determines our sleeping habits. I hope you can see clearly why this particular genetic pattern developed in our remote past. It is a survival instinct, pure and simple. And any understanding of insomnia needs to begin with this insight into the nature of our sleeping patterns.

One of the findings in insomnia research in the last couple of decades has been that insomnia almost always is associated with a disruption of one's sense of communal security and belonging. As long as we have at least one primal relationship with someone we sleep in the same house with, and as long as this relationship is not threatened one way or another, we tend to be able to sleep quite well. But as soon as something happens in our life, either emotionally or economically, which threatens our sense of ongoing communal security, we begin to experience an inability to relax into the ancient process of the nightly cycles of sleep.

In fact, separation or the threat of separation from

someone or some situation which has provided us with a communal feeling in life seems to be a prime generator of disturbed sleep patterns. There are many variations on this general theme, and of course some exceptions as well. But we will do well to look in this direction if we want to discover some of the sources of your insomnia.

Childhood Togetherness Memories

Before we move on to more specific discussions of sleeping and sleeplessness, I want to give you a chance to put the book aside for a few moments now, so you can look back at your childhood and remember the level of tribal togetherness you felt when going to sleep at night. In general did you sleep well as a child? And can you begin to remember how you felt as you drifted into sleep in your childhood bed?

CHAPTER ONE

Anatomy of a Good Night's Sleep

Throughout history there have been celebrated personalities who have thrived on very little sleep each night. Napoleon was said to sleep less than three hours a night, and yet was full of energy the next day. Chou En-lai was another leader who required only a few hours of sleep each night in order to wake up refreshed and ready for the next day. And the prolific genius and inventor Thomas Edison was famous for taking two or three short naps of less than an hour in order to gain all the sleep he needed every day.

So who can say how long we need to sleep, and what actually constitutes a good night's sleep? Sleep researchers have come to the conclusion, after studying many cases of people who need very little sleep, that the total time you spend with your eyes closed at night is not what is important to your waking up feeling refreshed. What is important is how much time you actually spend in delta sleep.

Delta sleep, as I mentioned in the introduction, is a special state of consciousness in which your mind lets go of thoughts and fantasies and relaxes completely. Your body also goes through a deep muscular relaxation during delta sleep, so that your entire system can rest in profound peace.

What people who need very little sleep are in fact doing when they sleep is this: they go almost immediately into delta sleep, rather than spending considerable time going step by step down into this deepest sleep state. And then when they come up out of delta sleep, they spend only a brief time, if any, in the dream phase of sleeping.

Thus, in less than an hour, they can obtain perhaps forty-five minutes of delta sleep. This is actually all the time the average person spends in delta sleep during an entire eight-hour slumber. Researchers don't know why a few people have such unusual sleep patterns; what we do understand is that they are getting enough of the essential type of sleep to refresh them for an entire day.

There is another key piece of sleep research which gives us insight into the nature of a good night's sleep. As you can see from the diagram at right, we do almost all of our delta sleeping during the first two sleep cycles of the night, which means during the first three hours of sleep. Later in the night, we simply don't drop down into delta sleep at all, but instead spend more time in lighter sleep and in dreaming.

What this means is that your first three hours of sleep are the most important for waking up refreshed in the morning. And when these first three hours are disturbed for one reason or another, even if you then sleep for twelve hours, you will not gain adequate amounts of delta sleep.

What do we learn from this? First of all, if you are a person who sleeps for a few hours and then wakes up and has a hard time getting back to sleep, perhaps you don't need to worry so much about the sleep you are losing during the early morning hours. You have probably already had enough delta sleep to completely satisfy you for the next day's activities.

Conversely, if falling asleep in the evening is your problem, then perhaps you should put off bedtime for an hour or two, or find a successful way to get to sleep soon after going to bed. If you suffer from nighttime insomnia but can fall asleep in a daytime nap, this is one way of gaining adequate delta sleep each day, until you resolve the causes of insomnia and learn techniques for getting to sleep easily in the evening.

Curiously, a good night's sleep can be ruined as easily by too much sleep as by too little. For several reasons which we will explore in their proper place, some people don't want to open their eyes and rise to the surface of consciousness after sleeping through the night. Instead, they stay in

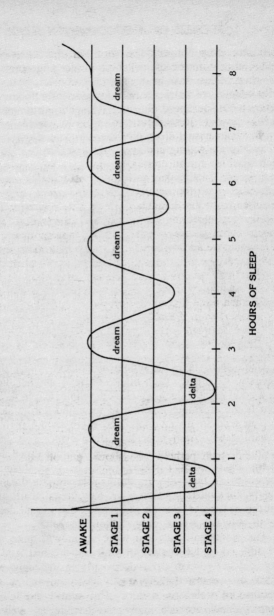

AWAKE

STAGE 1

STAGE 2

STAGE 3

STAGE 4

dream · delta · dream · delta · dream · dream · dream · dream

HOURS OF SLEEP

1 · 2 · 3 · 4 · 5 · 6 · 7 · 8

bed and sleep longer. The result of this oversleeping is grogginess, sometimes irritability, and a general lack of positive energy flow in the body.

It should be pointed out, however, that some people naturally sleep longer than the average eight hours a night. Albert Einstein habitually slept ten to twelve hours a night, and his mind certainly didn't seem groggy the next day.

The conclusion which sleep researchers have come to is that there is no set rule regulating how long an individual should sleep, and there are no set personality types which you can identify with different sleep cycles and lengths. Furthermore, it seems perfectly okay if your sleeping time varies considerably as different factors in your life alter. There are times when you are so excited about the coming day that you wake up fully refreshed after six or less hours of sleep. And there are those times when you oversleep a couple of hours and luxuriate in the added hours in bed.

The key factor in whether you had a good night's sleep is if you had enough delta sleep to replenish your vitality, and if you got out of bed when you were in an optimum state of alertness, rather than using sleep to avoid the new day.

Delta sleep is a physiological process which the body needs to experience each night. There is another dimension to a good night's sleep which is psychological in nature, and that is the dreaming function of the mind during sleep.

You tend to dream more and more as the night moves toward dawn. After your first sleep cycle, you dream for only about twenty minutes before heading down for delta again. But with each progressive cycle, your dreaming time increases, so that with the third cycle you are dreaming for nearly three-quarters of an hour. You dream nearly this long on the last two cycles as well, when there is no delta sleep at all between cycles, only shallow sleep.

The emotional state you wake up in will quite naturally be affected by the content of your last dreams. And even if you did get enough delta sleep early in the night, you can wake up exhausted, emotionally confused and in turmoil, because of traumatic dreams. I'm sure I am telling you nothing new—we all know the terrible as well as the beautiful effects our dreams can have on our feeling of rest or fatigue in the morning.

As we shall see step by step, the causes of insomnia when you are trying to fall asleep in the evening are usually intimately related with the causes of bad dreams later on in the night. So as we approach solutions to your insomnia, we will at the same time be exploring solutions to bad dreams if this is a chronic problem for you.

When we are unable to directly admit to and express certain feelings in our real life during the day, we seem to use dreams to release emotional pressures in fantasy form at night. From this psychoanalytical point of view, people who don't dream adequately during the night (waking up in early morning and not getting back to sleep till dawn) might be losing important psychic release through avoiding the dream states. If this is happening, then the loss of sleep/dream time will make it harder to deal with emotional struggles during the day.

The long-term solution to dreaming problems again lies with a conscious process of honest reflection on one's present life situation. I must say at this point that you must be somewhat of a champion if you are going to face the inner conflicts which are causing your insomnia, and deal with them directly. Sometimes people do need a little professional help to look honestly at themselves and see what changes need to happen in their lives, if they are to grow beyond the conflicts which underlie the sleep symptoms. Life isn't always easy.

But at the same time that I say this, I also feel the strong hope which I have developed through the years, based on seeing hundreds of people succeed in their struggle to break free of old habits and attitudes, and move forward into a satisfying new phase of their life. And it has been my experience that for every seriously disturbed person who must have some professional help in order to grow, there are hundreds of average people who can in fact help themselves, if only they are given the basic tools for making progress in their personal evolution.

Each paragraph I write will, I hope, generate a new piece of the puzzle you are seeking to solve, concerning what you need in order to help yourself through the phase of life you are presently in. You don't have to agree with what I am saying—what I hope is that you take in what I say, see if it rings bells for your personal situation, and take time to experiment with the various suggestions I will make. In this way we can cover most of the ground which we would explore if we were working together in person, so that you do gain direct contact with professional guidance in your quest for a good night's sleep.

Usually clients come to my office complaining about various emotional and physical symptoms that are bothering them so much that they are provoked into reaching out for help in relieving the symptoms. They can't get to sleep at night, for instance, and they want me to do something magical so that they do sleep. They see the particular symptom as the only problem they have. This is why people go to the doctor for sleeping pills when they suffer from insomnia.

Insomnia, however, is nothing more than a symptom. Something is keeping you awake—otherwise you would naturally drift into sleep according to your basic nature. So I challenge you to have the inner courage to start to look at what that "something" is which keeps you from falling asleep. I know that probably you have already done your best on your own to figure out what is causing your sleep-lessness. What I want to offer is some professional help based on an understanding of insomnia which you cannot be expected to have, since you are busy with your life and have not spent twenty years as a therapist looking at the problems that underlie the symptom of sleeplessness.

So if you provide the willingness to look, I'll provide the professional direction to your looking which is often needed to generate insight, personal growth, and a good night's sleep.

Before we move into a deeper look at the causes of insomnia, let me do what I will do at the end of every chapter, and give you a concrete technique to begin to learn for encouraging sleep.

I want to teach you a basic meditation which will stand as the central technique for the entire program. When I say *meditation*, by the way, I mean the word in purely secular terms, not in any particular spiritual tradition. Meditation means for me learning how to relax your mind, how to consciously turn off the chronic flow of thoughts, how to purposely guide your attention in directions you choose, which will benefit you.

All of us tend to be caught up in habitual flows of particular types of thoughts. We benefit from being able to think logically, of course. But we also suffer when our thinking minds dominate all the rest of our potential experience of life.

And this is certainly an important issue when it comes to insomnia, because almost always people who can't get to sleep are caught up in thinking about certain themes, in worrying about relationships or work or things done wrong in the past or terrible things that might happen in the future. It is our thoughts which tend to keep us awake, along with the resulting tensions and emotions in the body which are generated by those thoughts.

So a primary aim of this book is to teach you effective ways for quieting your thinking, worrying, problem-solving mind, so you can relax and sleep. Let me show you the basic mental-relaxation process, so you can begin to practice with it and make it your own. Practice is certainly the key to such shifts in awareness, by the way. The first few times you do this sleep-induction meditation, you probably won't be able to fully surrender to each step of the process. But in the next few nights, go through the ritual instead of lying awake wondering how to get to sleep.

And the good news is that for perhaps half of you, this primary sleep-induction method will prove to be all you need most of the time in order to gently progress from wakefulness into deep sleep. You can regularly practice the meditation when getting into bed, so that it becomes almost second nature every night. And you can certainly put it to use if you wake up in the middle of the night and need some help in getting back to sleep.

The Primary Sleep-Induction Meditation: Mind/Body Relaxation

The main object of this meditation is to gently move your awareness out of chronic thinking patterns and emotional contractions, and into a deeper awareness of your body here in the present moment. Shifting your attention toward finding good feelings to focus on in your body—this is one of the big steps to make in overcoming insomnia. And by adding to this basic shift in consciousness a simple sleep-inducing mental activity, you can quiet your mind, relax your body, and begin to drift into sleep.

I recommend that you read through the various phases of the meditation in order to gain an initial overview of the process. Then go back and do each phase, to begin to learn the actual experience of the meditation. Hold in mind that every time you do this sleep-induction process, you will have a new experience. You will feel your body relaxing in a unique way, and as you drift off into sleep.

1. Make sure that you are comfortable physically, by moving until your position feels just right. And begin to expand your awareness to include the sensation of the air which is rushing in and out your nose or mouth as you breathe. Don't make any effort to breathe, just let your inhales and exhales come and go as they want to, and tune into the feeling of the air coming and going through your nose or mouth. This simple shifting of your attention will prove very important in bringing you out of chronic thinking patterns and into an immediate awareness of yourself here in the present moment. Let your eyes close when they want to, so that your attention focuses more deeply on your breathing experience.

2. Along with the physical sensation of air rushing in and out through your nose and mouth, expand your awareness to include the physical movements in your chest, your belly, your rib cage and your back, which happen with every inhale and exhale. Breathing itself creates movement in your body, and by tuning into this present-moment feeling of the movement, you can bring yourself yet another step out of thoughts and into your body.

Learn to expand your awareness so that you can be aware of the sensation of air flowing in and out of your nose and mouth, and at the same time feel the movements in your body as you inhale and exhale.

3. Now to move gently one step deeper into relaxing your mind and body, expand your awareness to also include your jaw muscles. Usually when your mind is tense and restless, your jaw muscles will be tense as well. Consciously recognizing this habit of tension can very quickly help to relax your whole body. Let your jaw relax completely, as you stay aware of your breathing.

4. Now expand your awareness another step to include your pelvic region. Notice if you are holding those muscles down there tight, or if you are relaxed and feeling good in your pelvic and genital area. Insomnia very often provokes tense lower-back and pelvic muscles. Begin to relax these muscles by very gently moving your pelvis a bit with every breath. Rotate the pelvis back in its natural movement as you inhale, and then rotate it a little forward as you exhale. Relax your belly muscles as you inhale, and contract them a bit as you exhale. Do this breathing pattern a few times, and allow yourself to begin to feel good in your pelvic region.

5. Now relax your pelvic movements; be aware of how your body feels. Move your toes a little while you stay aware of your breathing. Tense and then relax your toes and legs, so that you feel good deep down in your feet and legs.

Move your fingers and hands a little, tensing and then relaxing them, so that a good flow of energy is felt in your hands and arms.

Go ahead and let your whole body move as it wants to now, to discharge any tensions in muscles everywhere in your body. Yawn if you want to, stretch, sigh, and let a beautiful rush of relaxation and good feelings flow through you with every new breath.

6. Now just relax completely. Stay aware of your breathing, of the sensation of air rushing in and out of your nose or mouth, and the movements in your body as you breathe. Surrender to a complete indulgence in the good feelings you have encouraged in your body. Say to yourself, "I'm ready for sleep . . ."

7. If you find yourself not quite drifting away into sleep at this point, simply begin to count your breaths as they come effortlessly one after the other. By saying the numbers to yourself, you will keep your mind busy so that thoughts won't begin to start up again. Say the number as you exhale slowly. And when you are at the bottom of each exhale, when there is a moment of no movement or airflow, say "Sleep" softly to yourself. Thus you exhale and say "One . . ." and then at the bottom of your exhale say "Sleep . . ." to yourself, then inhale with a beautiful silence inside you, then exhale and say "Two . . ." and then at the bottom of your exhale say "Sleep . . ." and so on until you drift into sleep. . . .

You now know a basic seven-step sleep-induction ritual which you can begin to practice, to memorize, so that each night you can go through the same routine, consciously moving your mind away from thinking and worrying while you move your body into relaxation and good feelings in the present moment. If you want extra assistance, there is a guided cassette program available for helping you surrender to the process. But you can also easily memorize the seven steps and take yourself off into sleep.

As I mentioned before, for many of you this basic sleep-induction process will be all you'll need, at least most of the time, to move from restlessness into a good night's sleep. The rest of the book will be dedicated to what to do when this is not enough. But each night before going to sleep, do spend time learning to surrender to each step of this seven-step process, so that you make it your own. And of course feel free to do any variations on the basic steps which you find enjoyable.

CHAPTER TWO

Too Many Sleepless Nights

In this chapter, I want to explore with you the different symptoms of insomnia, and then give you a technique for seeing to the heart of the sleep problems you are suffering from.

Losing a night or two of sleep because of a temporary trauma in your life is quite normal, and is not considered a form of insomnia at all. But when you have gone more than a few days, and less than a couple of weeks, without getting a good night's sleep, you are then medically considered a sufferer of what is labeled temporary insomnia. And when this condition extends beyond two weeks at a time without a break, you are said to suffer from chronic insomnia.

Sleep deprivation beyond a couple of nights has definite effects on your emotional condition. You experience frustration and anger at not being able to fall asleep. You feel a growing sense of panic and worry, because you know it is not good to go without sleep. And you feel hopelessness at your condition, mixed with dread of another sleepless night.

Sleep deprivation also causes reduced mental functioning the next day—concentration is noticeably lower, motivation is reduced, problem-solving ability is eroded, and a general reduction in learning ability occurs. When in experiments sleep deprivation is pushed into three or more days, subjects often begin to hallucinate, become easily angered even to the point of unwarranted violence, and begin to demonstrate paranoid behavior.

The inability to fall asleep at night is not a frivolous problem. You know that if you miss important sleep, you are going to do poorly at work. And this sets off a serious reaction of anxiety related to your very survival. What if you never get back to sleeping at night? What will become of you?

It is almost impossible to have insomnia and not to feel basic emotions of anxiety concerning your future and anger at your present condition. A therapist might see infinitely complex reasons for why you don't fall asleep at night, but there is no question about the resultant emotions that you suffer during sleepless nights. Many people even reach a state of complete mental confusion and emotional breakdown because of prolonged bouts of insomnia.

Unfortunately, worrying about whether you are going to be able to fall asleep the next night generates even more tension in your body, which continues to keep you from falling asleep. This is one of the most insidious traps for insomniacs, and we will explore several techniques for breaking free of it.

Curiously, although many people complain of not sleeping a single wink during the entire night, studies have shown that these "total" insomniacs are in fact sleeping as much as six or seven hours a night. What happens is this: they are sleeping lightly, but they are not experiencing delta sleep, and so their reports of not sleeping at all are physiologically correct—they have not spent any time at the level of sleep which brings rejuvenation to them, and so the next morning they feel as if they haven't slept a wink.

There are actually three types of insomnia. First of all, there is the variety where you can't get to sleep in the evening. Second, there is the experience of going to sleep in the evening, only to wake up several hours later and not be able to get back to sleep for an hour or two. And finally, there is the pattern of going to sleep and then waking up too early in the morning, and staying unhappily awake.

As I pointed out already, the first variety deprives you of your delta sleep; the second deprives you of perhaps the end of your delta and some of your dreaming time; and the third will interfere mostly with your final dreaming stages. If you are in top emotional shape, then the second two types of insomnia are not as serious as the first. But if there are strong disturbances inside you which are forcing you awake in order to avoid dreaming, then your suffering will be as great as the person who is losing early delta sleep.

Identifying Your Insomnia Type

Let's look for a few moments directly at your own recent experiences with insomnia. Pause and reflect about which type of insomnia you are suffering from, or which combination might best describe you.

1. Do you have difficulty with the first hours at night, when you want to fall asleep but are unable to?

2. Do you fall asleep in the evening, only to wake up suddenly a couple of hours later, and find it almost impossible to get to sleep afterward?

3. Do you sleep for four or five hours, but then wake up too early in the morning, wanting to get back to sleep but somehow wide awake long before the sun comes up?

Put this book aside for a few moments, and see what thoughts and insights, emotions and memories might be rising to the surface of your mind right now, related to your nighttime experiences.

The Insomnia Papers: Your Sleep Journal

To help you gain some valuable perspective on your restless, sleepless nights, it is important to start keeping a diary which records how you feel, what thoughts run through your head, and how your body feels while you are awake in the night. Are you worrying about a relationship crisis, for instance, or perhaps a problem at work? What in fact does go on inside you when you are having difficulties falling asleep?

What you remember of the night before when you get up the next morning is almost always inaccurate and hazy. But if you write down what is going on with you, right when it is happening, then the next morning you will find yourself reading extremely important facts about the actual nature of your insomniac bouts. And this interaction of your daylight consciousness and your nighttime consciousness will generate the insight you need in order to apply the techniques I am suggesting to you.

So please see if you can nightly write in your journal, expressing the thoughts, fantasies, emotions, and bodily sensations which are the ingredients of your sleeplessness. The following list is a general guideline to follow in exploring what aspects of your condition to write about.

Suggestions for Entries in Your Sleep Journal

a) Describe the main themes you think about at night:
   1) relationships
   2) past experiences
   3) future fantasies
   4) work
   5) problems to solve
   6) other thoughts
b) Describe the main emotions you feel at night:
   1) worry
   2) frustration/anger
   3) loneliness
   4) excitement
   5) grief/sorrow
   6) depression
   7) other emotions
c) Describe the fantasies you have at night:
   1) aggressive fantasies
   2) sexual desires
   3) an encounter with a friend
   4) horrible fantasies
   5) other fantasy themes
d) Once you have explored the above themes, writing whatever comes to mind, let yourself write about what you actually do, physically, during a bout with insomnia. Do you walk around the room pacing nervously, or perhaps sit despondently in a chair? Do you go eat everything in the refrigerator, or perhaps do exercises? Keep a good regular record in your

sleep journal of your habits of movement and activities when you are awake at night.

e) Also in your journal, keep a record of which exercises and meditations from this book you do, and how you respond to them. It's important to make these nocturnal notes, because you will tend to forget what happened when you wake up the next morning.

f) The final regular journal routine I suggest is that every morning after a bout of insomnia, you take a few minutes to read over what you wrote in your journal the night before, so that you can see clearly what the actual insomnia experience was, as well as your reaction to it. This reflective part of journal-keeping is very helpful in stimulating insight into what you might do in the future. Be sure to make notes the next morning of your reflections and ideas, so that there is a full circle to your journal.

Now that you have the basic structure of a sleep journal laid out for you, I strongly advise you to buy yourself a special notebook for this purpose, and to keep it by your bed. If you can develop the habit of writing in your journal every time you find yourself awake, you will be surprised at how the actual process of writing down your thoughts and feelings, your movements and activities will magically help to free you from your restlessness and get you back to sleep.

You can of course also use a tape recorder if this is your preference over writing. The important thing is that you regularly do make your entries, so that you gain an expanded perspective on what your insomnia actually consists of.

If you have pen and paper handy, you might want to take time right now to write down everything you can remember of what happened in your last bout with insomnia. Write down whatever comes to mind.

CHAPTER THREE

Primary Insomnia Sources

A funny thing happened to me on my way toward sunrise this morning. Suddenly I was wide awake and looking over at my clock, and the clock was looking back at me and saying three twenty-seven. I glanced outside and it was pitch-black. But my mind was already buzzing, my body tense and uncomfortable, and my emotions somehow agitated.

So early in the morning, my mind was already struggling to solve the problem of the new day—the writing of this challenging chapter in my insomnia book.

At the same time, I found myself caught up in an unfinished dream. I was dreaming about the first deep relationship which I formed after leaving home and losing close contact with my parents. I was madly in love with this girl, but then something went wrong and the affair ended. My dream was about this old romance. It was a terrible trauma as she stood up and fired a final rejecting glance in my direction, and then walked out the door.

Lying there in bed, awake, I was still caught in that feeling of excruciating hurt and humiliation at being left by my deepest love. The part of my mind wanted me to remember what happened to me during the weeks after she left me. But my raw emotional reaction was to totally shut those memories away. In fact, ever since that traumatic experience, I had avoided remembering what had happened to me alone in the world, without girlfriend, and without Mommy to run back to.

About an hour of very confused and traumatic time went by this morning as I lay suffering through an insomnia attack. I couldn't get back to sleep, that was for certain. And yet I couldn't throw off sleep and get up either.

In the midst of my racing thoughts I remembered my old habit of writing in my insomnia diary, and this thought stuck helpfully in my mind and gave me the motivation to get up and start writing.

I began to write about my dream first of all, and then about all the thoughts that had been buzzing around my mind for the last hour. And then I found myself writing down what had happened to me in reality after my girlfriend had left me.

The memories came tumbling over each other in their hurry to be recalled and released. I had in fact experienced a period of prolonged insomnia for the first time in my life. I was right in the middle of exams when the separation happened with my girlfriend; and there I was, unable to fall asleep at night even though I was desperately tired from cramming for exams. Night after night I would struggle to sleep, but somehow it was impossible until the early morning hours. And then I would sink into unconsciousness only to wake up late in the morning, cover my head, and sleep some more.

When I did finally get up out of bed, I was groggy, unable to concentrate. From my perspective now, I can say simply that I wasn't getting any delta sleep at all, and was suffering from sleep deprivation as a result. But from my perspective back then, I was going crazy, my entire life was falling apart, it was the end of the world.

Then a fortuitous event happened. I had been somewhat estranged from my parents for several years due to my involvement in the antiwar activities of the '60s, and contact with my mother had somehow been lost when I fell in love with my girlfriend. My girlfriend quite naturally took the place of my mother as the most important deep heart contact in my life.

Out of the blue one evening, about a week after my

separation from my girlfriend, my mother phoned me. She said she had just been wondering how I was doing, and I immediately began pouring out my tale of woe, even crying as I recounted my terrible situation. It was a great release of sorrow, grief, and anger, and my mother played the world's greatest therapist and kept relatively quiet while I relieved myself of my feelings.

Thanks to this honest relating, my mother and I felt our old contact again, and when I hung up the phone I felt that I wasn't alone anymore. And to be quite honest, I went to bed and slept like a baby all night. I talked with my mother and with my father also the next evening, and with this feeling of good old family unity radiating inside me again, I was able to work through my romantic problems success- fully, and was at least temporarily free of insomnia attacks.

I hope you forgive me for indulging in telling my personal account of insomnia blues, but my story represents what I want to discuss with you in this chapter. Although there are a number of causes of insomnia, the most common—the one which afflicts most people who develop non–drug-related insomnia—is the trauma of separation, in one form or another.

Psychiatrists call this condition separation anxiety. It has been my long-term observation with clients who come to me complaining of sleep disorders that this is the underlying cause of sleeplessness, and the professional journals also attest to this.

Surprisingly, most sufferers from insomnia do not recog- nize separation anxiety as the source of their problem. Let me go back to my own story a moment, to point out my own failings in this regard.

Like almost all of you, I grew up in a supportive family, felt cozy in bed at night like a Hottentot in the tribal circle of sleeping heads. And like most children, I was quite dependent on my parents, especially my mother, for that primal feeling of well-being and acceptance. When I went to college and began to break free of my childhood depen- dency on my family circle, I quickly found someone new to be dependent on emotionally, someone who would see me with loving eyes, accepting my entire personality (even though there were parts to it that were in serious need of improvement).

Then when I lost my new relationship and found myself all alone in the world, I was gripped by a terrible anxiety. For the first time in my life I was totally alone. What a terrible experience! And in that solitary condition, my habits of sleeping were violated. Sleep for me was a communal experience. But then there I was in bed alone, in an empty house, with a number of friends but no primary relationship to hold on to as I drifted into sleep.

So drift I could not. It was that simple.

Over the years I have grown more mature, so that I find more of my security within myself and place less on the shoulders of other people. This is what maturity is all about—becoming more independent, while still keeping one's heart open to deep relationships.

But back when that first separation trauma grabbed me, I was in no position to admit to myself or to friends that I was in reality still a mama's boy who couldn't survive in the world without the security of a trusting relationship there with me either in the flesh or in fantasy projections.

I later learned to live happily alone for periods of time, and thus overcame the trauma of standing on my own two feet—or more precisely of sleeping in my own solitary bed. But I am still most happy when I have a strong primary relationship in my life, and I find myself happily married as a consequence.

But enough of me—what about you? Please don't think that I expect you to project my experience onto your unique life. Quite the opposite, in fact. I want you to see if your bouts with insomnia come from a different source than mine did. Let's consider other causes of insomnia, and see when bells ring in your own situation.

1. Many people suffer from sleepless nights simply because they drink several cups of coffee during the day as a regular habit. *Caffeine* will quite powerfully keep you awake at night, even if you are sleeping in your true love's arms without a separation worry in sight.

Many *prescription medications* can do the same, as we will explore in more detail in the next chapter. In fact, almost always when people try to give up medications, their sleep is disturbed for a period of time while the body adjusts to the removal of the drugs from the system. So perhaps your sleeping problem is drug-related. Certainly if you use *cocaine* you will find sleep a difficult experience, to say the least, and the same is true of *mood elevators* and *diet pills* and the like.

2. Another common cause of insomnia is *environmental stress*. In plain terms this means the guy in the apartment above you who plays loud music all night, or the dog that barks through the wee hours, or the couple fighting it out next door when you're trying to get some shut-eye.

Temporary insomnia certainly can be generated by *noise pollution* of many kinds, but it should be pointed out that most people quickly learn to filter out such noises as they go to sleep, and are relatively unbothered in the long run even by jets taking off right over their heads all night. But if you have other reasons for insomnia, then your mind will latch onto environmental disturbances and blame them for the entire sleep difficulty you are experiencing.

3. *Pain* can also be a cause of chronic or temporary insomnia. Any health problem that has a physical symptom will tend to upset your sleep; I deeply sympathize with this condition, having known it well myself at times. Hopefully the programs in this book will be of help if pain is a primary cause of sleepless nights. But I also ask you to be open to the possibility that pain is not the only cause of your insomnia.

4. *Stress at work* can definitely keep one awake at night. If there is uncertainty in your life related to your financial well-being, then the resultant *anxiety* will very often generate insomnia.

Many people attach themselves to their work situation in the same way they would to a lover or mate or parent. We all seem to need to be a part of some tribal organization to one extent or another. It's human nature to move through life with a sense of relationship with the culture around us, since our survival ultimately depends on our participation in our extended tribal system.

It is very common these days to find people who have their primary bonding not with a single person, but with a group of people at work, and in fact with the company or organization itself. They feel a part of something greater than themselves, they feel accepted, they feel safe and secure in the hands of their employer. Thus when fear of losing a job is raised, separation anxiety comes into being just as surely as if your spouse or lover threatens to leave you.

It is important to treat the fear of losing a job, or the actual loss of a job, with the same seriousness as the threat or loss of a significant emotional relationship. In fact, any anxiety related to failure in life will evoke the conditions that cause insomnia. Students afraid of failing exams often experience bouts of insomnia which go away once the exam is finished and passed.

5. In the old days, there was one punishment a tribe or community could order which was in fact experienced by the unfortunate recipient of the punishment as a fate perhaps worse than death itself: *expulsion* from the tribe. Traditionally, a person expelled or exiled from his lifetime relationship with his community was a hopeless, tormented soul, wandering the earth with no place to rest.

I believe we still carry within us this primal fear of rejection and abandonment. People who are caught up in separation anxiety are in fact the majority of people who suffer from insomnia. The separation can be from your wife or husband or lover, or from your work or school or even your prison. I remember working at San Quentin, a high-security prison in California, for a short time. I was helping convicts adjust to life on the inside of the prison, and also helping newly released convicts to adjust to the outside world. And in both cases, going into prison *and* leaving prison, there was almost always a period of sleep disturbance related to being separated from familiar environment and friends.

And of course, the ultimate separation anxiety is that of facing death itself. When children first begin to realize that they are mortal beings, they quite naturally experience a temporary period of traumatic sleep while the psyche attempts to deal with the inevitable reality of permanent separation from this entire life we are so attached to. Throughout one's lifetime, there are recurring periods of sleepless nights as the reality of our coming death hits on deeper and deeper levels.

In your own personal situation, what is keeping you from having a good night's sleep these days? Are you caught up in the anxiety and agony of fearing rejection, separation, isolation, banishment from a person or situation you need? Have you already lost someone you need in your life in order to relax and go to sleep? Are you afflicted by pain that won't let you sleep, or by noise pollution? Are you chronically taking drugs of one type or another that are ruining your nighttime surrender into a good long sleep? Is your work stress jamming your mind all the time, so that you simply cannot turn your thoughts off and drift into sleep? Or is there some other cause for your present lack of relaxation and sleep? Take a few important moments now to put the book aside, breathe, relax a bit, and see what comes to mind.

It is true that many people look to their present lives for a cause of separation anxiety, but seem to find none at all. Very often insomnia hits us out of the blue, and on the surface we can find absolutely no reason for it.

One of the thrills of being a therapist is playing the mystery game of searching for the hidden cause of a physical symptom like insomnia. Often it takes only one or two sessions to find the experience which stimulated separation anxiety and the bout of insomnia. Even a friend talking with you, after reading this book, can probably help you to come to the realization of the source of your trauma.

For instance, I remember a client who was happily in love with his wife, secure in his profession, healthy, and quite a bright friendly fellow. But two weeks before I first saw him, he was suddenly hit with insomnia attacks that threatened to tear his whole life apart through sleep deprivation. He took no drugs, had no strange hidden compulsions. He just was unable to fall asleep at night.

So we went back to the days immediately before the insomnia hit him, and began our investigation of everything that happened to him. In a fairly short time, he was talking about the fact that his father had phoned him around the time he started losing sleep, but it had been an unimportant conversation and he couldn't recall the contents of the discussion.

I had him pause long enough to bring the phone call more clearly into focus. His father had talked of many things, but had briefly mentioned that his wife, my client's mother, was going into the hospital for a checkup soon. It was just a statement that went by and was gone, as more pressing discussions of a mutual business transaction were worked through.

But my client, upon remembering this forgotten bit of information, was suddenly trembling. He was a big man who was not used to crying in front of other men I am sure, but there were definite tears welling up inside him as he realized he had pushed the news of his mother going into the hospital completely out of his mind, and hadn't even called back to see what the results of the exam had been. His unconscious mind, however, had apparently taken this possible question of his mother's health quite seriously indeed.

From my office he called his mother, and had a good heart-touching talk with her, finding out that there had been no medical difficulties discovered in her exam at all, so there was no need to worry. He was greatly relieved, and with this hidden threat to his relationship with his mother uncovered and resolved, he had no further trouble in sleeping during that point in his life.

But when his mother did fall ill several years later, his insomnia recurred; he did have a difficult time going through the trauma of her resultant death, as most of us do when we experience the final separation from a loved one.

Sometimes the detective work in exposing the causes of insomnia can be quite simple, but sometimes it takes longer. And of course, sometimes causes are complex and buried under many years of accumulated memories. What I challenge you to do at this point is to begin looking into your past, to see if you can discover what happened to generate the insecurity and anxiety, the sense of uncertainty and nervousness, the frustration and the hostility as well, which keep you from falling asleep. Let me give you a beginning meditation to get you started.

Insomnia Detective Work

If you are suffering from insomnia, take five minutes each night when you are unable to sleep, and five minutes sometime during the day, and do the following meditation.

Relax a moment, tune into your breathing, and ask yourself this question: what has happened in your life to make you feel restless and insecure, emotionally upset and physically tense?

Notice how your body feels. Notice the tensions in your breathing. And without effort, begin to allow memories to come to mind, either of the recent past or further back, which might shed light on the state of nervous agitation which keeps you from sleeping at night.

If you feel emotional pressures building up inside you as you search for the causes of your insomnia, be sure to breathe through the mouth, and open yourself to whatever emotions might want to flow up and out of you. In the middle of such emotional flows often come sudden insights into the source of your sleeplessness.

Keep your insomnia journal handy and make notes about what memories and ideas come to you, even if they seem unrelated to your sleepless condition. All clues are valuable!

Each time you repeat this "detective" meditation, you will find yourself going deeper in directions which might offer the solution to your dilemma. When you think you have found a clue or even the answer to your search, write down what you have discovered, but don't necessarily think that your discovery is correct—your mind will sometimes play games with you.

What is important is that you regularly point your attention in this detective-memory direction, so that you are activating deep reflective processes which stimulate intuitive insight. Trust your intuitive self, go on an adventure, and get to know yourself better in the process!

CHAPTER FOUR

The Great Sleeping Pill Hoax

A person walks into his doctor's office complaining of insomnia. The doctor looks across his desk and sees a human being who is obviously suffering from lack of sleep and related emotional and mental traumas. In all fairness to most doctors, the first thought that probably crosses the doctor's mind is that this person should see a therapist and get some direct help in resolving the causes of the insomnia. Doctors know full well that insomnia is almost always just a symptom, not a disease in itself.

But most doctors end up simply prescribing sleeping pills instead of professional counseling for their patients with insomnia. Why is this so? First of all, doctors often suggest therapy to their patients, only to have the patients resist the idea of going to a "shrink" for a simple problem with sleeping. Therapists are expensive, furthermore.

Doctors also hesitate to suggest therapy for their insomnia patients because doctors in general are not well-trained in dealing with emotional causes of illness, and traditionally have resisted the very notion of psychosomatic dimensions to disease. It is only in recent years that the importance of emotional health has been included in medical treatment strategies.

Sometimes, of course, you are lucky enough to go to a doctor who has both the time and the psychological understanding to help you directly with the resolution of your insomnia condition. You tell him or her you are having trouble falling asleep, and then the two of you talk for an hour or so about your problems, and perhaps you come back several times for more counseling. This would be ideal, but unfortunately our health system is so greatly pressured by time constraints that almost no doctor can take that much time for each patient, even if he or she wants to and knows how to help people in non-drug situations.

So almost always, after just a brief discussion of the nature of insomnia, the doctor writes out a prescription, the patient takes it to the drugstore, and a very serious step is made in the history of that patient.

I know that many of you who are reading this book are already involved with sleeping pills and other types of mood-altering medications. I don't want to make you feel that your doctor has done something bad to you in prescribing drugs for your insomnia condition. From a medical point of view, this is perfectly reasonable and proper procedure. You go to the doctor for treatment of some kind for your condition, and apart from therapy, the only treatment medically available for insomnia is in fact drugs—along with a few suggestions about not drinking coffee and trying to work through your personal problems on your own.

We must hold in mind that the tools of medical practitioners are very basic—doctors administer drugs, and doctors perform surgery. They work with myriad amazing drugs, of course, and they can do miracles with surgery these days. But except for some basic advice offered to you during a treatment session, doctors are limited to the above two avenues for helping you. Being a doctor can be a frustrating job, because they see so much suffering and yet they have only their limited ways of alleviating the suffering. By and large, medical treatment is aimed at relieving symptoms, and very often does not reach down to the underlying causes of chronic disease.

So when you go to your doctor and are given sleeping pills to help you deal with your insomnia, the doctor's logic is this: you are suffering from a symptom caused by emotional conflicts. The medication will give you relief from serious loss of delta sleep, and in the meanwhile you will hopefully be able to resolve your emotional problems on your own and return to normal sleeping patterns.

In many instances, this logic is correct. People usually do recover from painful loss and separation from loved ones on their own. And yes, there are definitely times when sleeping pills are helpful in softening the blow of grief and depression. I myself recommend sleeping pills at times to clients, when administered carefully for limited periods of time.

But as all too many of you know from personal experience, the simple reality is that all sleeping pills are habit-forming. Many of them are physically addictive, and all of them are psychologically addictive. This is serious business we are talking here. The evening news is filled with the anger of the populace against dealers in such drugs as cocaine and heroin. But the same citizens who are crying out for the arrest and even the execution of drug dealers are stopping by the drugstore to pick up their new prescriptions for Amytal, Seconal, Dalmane, Luminal, Tranxene, Miltown, Librium, Elavil, Tofranil, and so on. Many of these prescription drugs are strongly addictive, lethal in overdose, and potentially just as destructive to long-term users as are the black-market drugs we fear so much.

Basically, we should be clear about the fact that there as yet exists no prescription drug which simply puts you to sleep. The drugs that are labeled "sleeping pills" work only through affecting your entire central nervous system. They are knockout drugs. Rather than leading you into the natural stages of restful sleep, sleeping pills override the natural sleep cycles and push you into a very different unconscious experience, in which normal delta sleep is never replicated.

Therefore you wake up in a drugged condition the morning after using a sleeping pill. Perhaps you have not had to suffer from the emotional trauma of a sleepless night, but you have definitely not experienced your natural sleep cycles either. You have been comatose, your central nervous system sufficiently stunned to induce sleep, but not so much as to turn you off completely and kill you. Medical experts do know the proper dosages which take you under without doing you in. But there is no pill which induces natural sleep.

Not only is your relationship with delta sleep disturbed with sleeping pills—your relationship with your entire inner dream world is of course seriously distorted as well. Much of your dreaming is simply drugged out of existence. And the dreams which you have under the influence of a knockout drug are very different, to say the least, from what you would otherwise experience.

As a further problem with pill-taking, there is always the challenge of breaking free of your drug dependency sometime in the future. The unfortunate fact is that when you stop taking drug treatment for insomnia, your insomnia almost always returns, usually much more severely. Thus you have gained nothing in the long run from taking your pills, but instead have been set back in your condition noticeably. It is very hard to "come off" sleeping pills, regardless of whether you do it gradually, as most doctors recommend, or simply throw the damned bottle away and go "cold turkey." You *can* stop using them, but only after suffering through withdrawal.

There is certainly a minority of you reading this book who do need help from sleeping pills and mood elevators for maintaining your stability in the present moment. I am not suggesting that all of you throw away your prescriptions and face tonight on your own. Certainly there are times for temporary medical help.

What I am advocating in this book is the urgent need to move toward a drug-free sleeping experience as soon as possible, if in fact you are presently dependent on drugs for nightly sleep. Life is simply too short to spend it in a drugged state, don't you agree?

I suspect that you started taking sleeping pills simply because you were suffering; you were almost in a panic because of your sleepless condition—and sleeping pills were the only available treatment you could find to help relieve your symptoms. The habit of popping sleeping pills has become so commonplace that we tend to do it almost automatically, assuming that if everybody else is doing it, then it must be okay.

But ask any doctor—problems are manifold and almost universal among pill users. There is no safe sleeping pill. They all make you dependent on them. When insomniacs move from sleepless nights to drug-induced sleep, they are moving from a natural problem with emotional dependency to a chemical problem with drug dependency. Instead of having a human friend whom they depend on for the security which leads to good sleep, they have substituted a drug.

In both cases, we should note clearly, the problem lies in not having yet moved forward in life to a more independent state, where the security needed to fall asleep is found within.

These are difficult words for me to be saying to those of you who are presently dependent on drugs for your nightly sleep. But there is no other way I can find to express these harsh realities. If you are presently dependent on sleeping pills, mood elevators, tranquilizers, pep pills, diet pills, or any of the other "miracle pills" which have come onto the market, I can only say this: do whatever you can to break the habit. Use the techniques you are learning in this book first of all, and see if you can get free of drug dependency on your own. Go to your doctor and tell him your intent of quitting drugs, and ask his advice on the best procedure for reducing your present prescription. And if you cannot stop on your own, then contact a good drug-rehabilitation center where you can gain expert guidance on your way to a drug-free future.

This is a great challenge, I know. I have had two bouts with similar drug-dependency situations myself, and as I write this challenge to you, I know full well the ordeal you might have to go through to get clean again. But I am sure you know in your heart that being dependent on drugs is no way to go through life, if there is even a spark of hope that you can move beyond drugs into a new brighter future.

It is an absolute travesty that as we grow older we almost invariably begin taking more and more drugs just to get through the day. I cannot help but cry out against our present medical situation, in which we are placing the vast majority of our research money into the development of yet more drug treatments for almost every symptom you can imagine.

It is a hoax that drugs can cure us of all our problems. Drugs treat *symptoms*. And for every symptom relieved, a side effect from the drug is usually brought into play which will further disrupt the natural equilibrium of health.

In reality there is no chemical solution to emotionally caused conflicts and symptoms. We must ultimately have the courage to face our own selves, to admit what is bothering us, and then take the realistic steps which are required for growth and improvement to occur in our lives. What I am trying to do is to offer you the professional tools which can greatly ease the growth pains, and help you to move as rapidly as possible toward regaining your balance in life.

But very little emotional growth can occur when you are in a drugged state. This is a reality of life. You have to come out of the numbed state induced by sleeping pills, you have to feel directly the agony of grief and isolation, of anger and frustration, if you are to move through these emotions and into a new period of joy and peace.

Let's end this chapter with a powerful meditation which I recommend you do regularly if you are presently using sleeping pills and would like to break the habit. If twice a day you do this imaginary exercise of clearing your home and body of drugs, you will consciously reprogram your attitudes and habits in the direction of a drug-free future. Memorize the exercise so you can guide yourself through it; also step by step reduce your nightly dosage of sleeping chemicals, and your daily doses of whatever you might be taking for mood elevators and relaxants.

The Beyond-Drugs Meditation

Relax for a few moments, make yourself comfortable, and close your eyes when you feel ready. Stretch and yawn if you feel any tensions in your body, and tune into your breathing as each breath comes and goes effortlessly.

Now begin to imagine that you no longer use drugs to help you through the days and nights. Imagine that you have broken free of drug dependencies for your emotional stability, and moved into a new expansive period in your life where you are free from chemical distortions of your awareness.

Imagine that there are no drugs at all in your medicine cabinet or anywhere else in your house. You have thrown all the old prescriptions out, and cleaned up your environment so that no traces of your former dependent habits remain. Look all over your house where you used to keep your pills, and see that you are free of these pills now, that they no longer exist in your world.

Imagine that, every day, you eat healthy food. Your body is thriving on an optimum diet. You are also getting plenty of exercise, and your body feels happy again like it did when you were younger.

And imagine that when you go to bed tonight, you can relax, calm your thoughts and emotions, feel secure in your own heart, and drift into a beautiful night's sleep . . .

Of course in reality this might not be the case as yet, but by imagining such an ideal life, you point your inner self in the right direction, so that the actual steps toward a drug-free, sleep-full life will be much easier to make. The meditation only takes a few minutes to do, and it can prove extremely powerful in bringing about changes in your life. Go for it!

CHAPTER FIVE

Sleeping Like a Baby

What an extraordinarily beautiful experience it must have been for all of us as we floated in perfect peace and security for so many months in our mother's womb, with all our worldly needs taken care of, and with no anxiety or insecurity to disturb our blissful existence.

But then the perfect bliss came to an abrupt and traumatic end, as we grew too big for the inner sanctity of the womb, and were unceremoniously pushed out into a harsh world of gravity and air and an ongoing struggle to take care of our separate selves in the world.

Life is an inexorable progression from our original security and oneness with our mother into a more and more separate, independent, solitary condition, and our challenge is to mature step by step toward finding our sense of security within ourselves, not in those around us.

But even as we mature we should be able to regularly slip into the ultimate state of relaxation and trust we knew when we used to fall asleep as babies and small children. I am blessed with a new baby son these days, and I continue to marvel at this spontaneous ability to move into delta sleep which all babies are born with.

You were almost certainly such a baby yourself, able to tap effortlessly into the eternal peace of delta sleep whenever your biological batteries needed recharging and rest. And in your childhood years also, you probably had an easy time falling asleep and sleeping peacefully through the night.

I wonder if you can remember bedtime when you were young? Can you picture your little bed, your special blanket which you curled up under, a teddy bear or doll perhaps? And can you remember the final soothing words spoken to you, the gentle good-night kiss which let you know that you would be watched over while you slept, so that you could relax and trust completely in a safe night of sleep?

In my work with clients suffering from insomnia, I almost always include sessions which help them to go back, back, back into their early childhood, so that they can remember the peace of childhood sleep, and regain that special sense of bliss and calm which is lacking in their present sleep routines. How do you feel about going back into your childhood days and nights, to make new contact with your successful sleep patterns?

In order to do this, you will need to practice the age-regression process I am going to teach you, so that step by step memories begin to open up to you.

Please keep in mind that many people, especially people who are suffering from insomnia, at first have a somewhat difficult time in turning their attention toward childhood experiences. In fact, it is precisely this sense of estrangement from positive early-childhood feelings that lies at the heart of insomnia. Life has not been easy for us as we moved into adulthood and all its resultant frustrations and separations from those we loved. And we tend to lose that special childhood sense of trustful peace, that state of eager anticipation of the bliss of slipping into yet another night's sleep.

But you can begin to regain that early experience of a good night's sleep. Quite possibly this chapter will be a vital key in your quest for a non-drug sleeping remedy. I must confess that it is certainly one of my own ways of falling asleep at night. If I'm addicted to anything, it is to a nightly return to that immensely satisfying feeling that I knew as a youngster. I hope you can quickly learn to regain this feeling as well.

The Age-Regression Experience
(Early Childhood Memories)

You can imagine practicing this technique while reading these pages. Please hold in mind that if you are using sleeping pills, their influence will make this process more difficult to do—and hopefully as you reduce your consumption of nightly medication, you will find a noticeable increase in your ability to move into your childhood states of sleep.

I have already taught you the beginning steps in this procedure. You lie in bed, on your back if this is comfortable, and turn your attention to your breathing, so that you begin to shift out of your thoughts and into your experiential mode of consciousness, i.e., the sensations you feel as you breathe. As you tune into your breathing in the present moment, also become aware of the tensions in your jaw muscles, and let them relax with every new breath. . . . Move your toes, and then your fingers as well, to release any tensions you find. . . . Also move your pelvis a little with every breath, to let a pleasurable rush flow through your body. . . . And then let yourself surrender to a good stretch and a couple of deep yawns, so that your physical body is moving in the direction of peaceful sleep, and your mind is relaxing its habitual flow of thoughts. . . .

Now roll onto your side for a few moments, and curl up in a comfortable position. We all have rituals of rolling and tossing and turning before we fall asleep. Let yourself surrender to a comfortable position which you also used to sleep in as a child. The fetal position of being curled up on your side is certainly an important one to explore.

In this position, begin to open yourself to feeling how you used to feel as a little boy or girl in bed, when you were finished with the day and ready for a good night's sleep.

Feel the bed under you, the blankets over you, and let yourself remember how it felt in your childhood bed, with your covers over you. Surrender to memories of being young, of being ready to go to sleep in your own little comfy spot in your family home. You have nothing to do, nowhere to go, you are relaxing into that beautiful blissful bodily feeling of complete pleasure, as thoughts drift away, and warm quiet perfect peace begins to fill your body. . . .

As you drift into sleep, you regress back into very infantile feelings, as if you are again curled up in the womb, safe, quiet, indulging in pure relaxation, drifting away into the infinite bliss of delta sleep. . . .

We were all brought up with regular reminders that we should let go of our babyhood, stop indulging in infantile feelings, and mature into grown-up adults. This is of course true—but there is at least one time in our day when it is essential to put aside all our maturity, to turn off our adult minds, and in fact indulge completely in our infantile feelings.

Bedtime is our chance to let go of everything, to just turn off all worries and responsibilities, and drift into the sleep we knew as a baby. Remember that until you were a year or two old, you did no real thinking at all—your mind was constantly, effortlessly always here in the present moment. This is why the consciousness of a baby is so close to the consciousness of a spiritual master—they are both living right here in the present moment all the time, not victims of chronic thoughts and worrying.

I just took time a few minutes ago to go upstairs and play with my nine-month-old son as he was getting tired and ready for his morning nap, and I am still luxuriating in how good it felt to hold him in my arms as he started to let go of waking reality and drift into sleep. What a beautiful human ability this is, this surrender to sleep!

You were once a baby like my little son, you once could fall asleep in your father's or mother's arms, or in your little bed, and drift off into that bliss of undisturbed rest and rejuvenation. Ah, it felt so good, to lie in your bed when you were little, to feel safe and sound under your warm blanket, trusting the universe to carry on while you let go and drifted away.. . . .

Why don't you give yourself a few moments right now to close your eyes and see what early memories come to you of the feeling of your childhood bed, the comfort of your covers over you, the secure aura of being with your family in your house. Your thoughts are quiet, the house is quiet, your jaw muscles relax, your pelvis relaxes, your whole body begins to melt into a delicious movement into sleep. You stretch one final time, yawn, and sigh. . . . Remember the bliss of slipping into deep slumber, and bring your childhood sleep habits back into your present life, so you sleep like a baby.

CHAPTER SIX

What Happens As We Grow Older

To tap back into the feelings and rituals we knew as young-sters, which worked so well to help us slip into deep sleep, is certainly a wise approach to inducing a good night's sleep. We do know how to go through the falling-asleep process by surrendering to the nonverbal process we were masters of when we were very young.

But it is also a fact that as we grow older, our sleep cycles begin to change, and recent sleep research has given us quite a clear picture of what these changes are. Perhaps most dramatic is the change in the amount of time we spend down deep in delta sleep.

The average twenty-year-old will drop into delta sleep for perhaps forty-five minutes or so a night, mostly during the first few hours of sleep. But as this person gets older, the number of minutes spent in delta sleep decreases noticeably.

The biological reasons for this reduction in delta sleep time are not understood, but the statistical facts stare us in the face, begging acceptance as a main cause of nocturnal disturbances as we grow older. By the age of sixty, delta sleep time is often reduced to just a few minutes a night. Many older people complain that the older they become, the less time they sleep each night. But this does not seem to be true. What does seem to be happening is that the experi-ence of sleep is changing, as just noted, so that deep sleep is not so plentiful.

Again back to statistics: on the average a person who is

twenty years old sleeps a total of four hundred and fifty minutes each night, while a person who is seventy sleeps a total of four hundred and forty. Ten minutes' difference in the sleeping time of these two age groups who are fifty years apart is simply not significant. So the claims of the elderly that they sleep less than they used to must be viewed in terms which are not specifically related to minutes spent asleep.

What actually seems to be happening is this: as we grow older, we tend to sleep a lighter sleep, spending much more time in stages one and two, rather than in three and four. (See chart on page 11.)

We also tend to wake up many more times when we are older than when we are young. When we are five, we might reach the point of wakefulness three or four times a night, during which we rise to the surface of sleep and just for a moment are conscious. But as we get older, these moments of wakefulness progressively increase, so that when we are fifty we are poking our heads into momentary wakefulness maybe thirty times a night; and this number climbs to sixty to a hundred brief wakenings per night as we become quite old.

So when someone over fifty says that he or she doesn't sleep much at night, this is a subjectively true statement, though it may not be objectively valid. It certainly *feels* to this person that less sleep was experienced, because the quality of the sleep has changed.

Along with the reduction in delta sleep, older people also complain of multiple physical symptoms such as aches and pains, frustration over lack of deep sleep, and downright anger about the loss of peace they once knew through sleep.

With most people bothered by sleep disturbances, however, the primary disturbance is not a physiological problem but an emotional one. People wake up in the middle of the night, or can't fall asleep at the beginning of the night, and begin worrying about the consequences of this loss of sleep—and the worrying itself becomes the main problem of the sleep disturbance, not lost sleep or recurrent awakenings.

Of course, as people grow older, there are often additional emotional traumas which exacerbate the natural changes in the sleep cycles. It is almost inevitable that the older we get, the more we must deal with a sense of aloneness and isolation, for instance. We begin to drift out of the mainstream of our cultural involvement as we retire from work and our children grow up and leave us alone after all those years of family life. And when our friends around us start to die, we are often left with feelings of grief, isolation, and painful loneliness.

Each of us has this final phase of life to move through, and it is our success in maturing through each previous stage of life which determines whether old age will be a beautiful culminating phase of a full life, or whether this final stage is beset with emotional trauma and despair.

I am only forty-three as I write this chapter, and thus will not pretend to preach about something which I have not as yet experienced personally. But I have worked with many clients over sixty, and from this work I hope to shed at least a little helpful light on the question of aging and sleeping.

One of the most important suggestions I make to elderly people, and in fact to anyone over twenty, is to begin to loosen up youthful concepts of how our individual nights should progress. We tend to be creatures of habit, and when it comes to sleeping, we expect each night to follow the same course as the ones before. But this is simply not how life progresses. Each night is unique, and if we get upset when our routine is altered, then we add unnecessary trauma to our sleep experience.

Instead, see if you can accept in a positive manner the variations which occur in your sleeping habits. When you suddenly wake up in the middle of the night and can't get back to sleep, don't panic. There are nights when it is perfectly normal to get out of bed, sit quietly in the living room, or even put on an overcoat and go for a midnight or early-morning walk.

If you always fight wakefulness when it comes to you in the middle of the night, you are causing yourself terrible frustration which is not called for. Who says that the middle of the night is only for sleeping! Perhaps there is a deep wisdom within you which wakes you up at particular points in a particular sleep cycle so that you can gain a special insight which is rising up in your unconscious at that moment.

I have already pointed out that after the first three hours of sleep you have gained all the delta sleep you are going to receive that night anyway. So why toss and turn trying to get back to sleep, when you don't need to? Why not open yourself to a unique nighttime experience instead?

Many elderly people come to this realization on their own. If you are over fifty you almost certainly know that there can be a special beauty in the middle of the night, if you open yourself to being awake instead of trying to force yourself to go back to sleep. The middle of the night, when accepted as a part of one's waking experience, can be a most rewarding time full of quiet peace, of deep meditation, of unexpected reflection and memories, and even sudden insights into problems which have not resolved themselves through daytime thinking.

So I encourage you to break free of those instant panics and reactions of frustration when you suddenly pop into wakefulness in the middle of the night. Trust your inner guide to bring you something unexpected and rewarding during the time you are awake. And then see if you return to bed and sleep after you have explored whatever experience comes to you while awake.

In many spiritual traditions, there is special emphasis placed on the hours between four A.M. and sunrise. The Essene tradition which Jesus seems to have spent time in, for instance, suggested that spiritual devotees wake up every morning at three-thirty, so that they could sit quietly and meditate from around four o'clock until the sun comes up.

This particular time of the day is considered in spiritual circles throughout the world to have a special power, a particular energy which is much weaker at all other times of the day. There exists an opportunity for spiritual clarity and insight at this time which is simply not to be found at other times of the day, according to Tibetan Buddhist tradition, American Indian tradition, ancient Egyptian tradition, and so on.

So when you suddenly are awake at four in the morning, you can either traumatize yourself through rejecting this wakefulness, or you can bless yourself by getting up, putting on some warm clothes if necessary, and sitting quietly during this special period, experiencing new feelings and insights that come to you, and enjoying being awake while the rest of the world is still sleeping.

Very often, people report to me that they get up at this time of the day, and then an hour or two later go back to bed for a final sleep cycle—and then get up feeling more refreshed than if they had slept through the whole night. This is my experience as well. I am not a fanatic in waking myself up each morning to meditate. But when I wake up spontaneously at an early hour, I take advantage of the time for a special experience at the beginning of the new day.

We should also consider the universal phenomenon of the afternoon nap in this context. Almost all babies take a nap in the afternoon, and this habit continues for many children until school begins to interfere with the routine. To drop into a single sleep cycle in the afternoon, and then to rise up for the duration of the day—this is such a beautiful routine that young ones are allowed to indulge in.

Many cultures encourage a continuation of this habit into adult life—i.e., the siesta found throughout warm climates. In these cultures people wake up early to work and play before it gets hot. Then they take a good long nap while the midday heat is pounding down outside. And then they stay up quite late at night to enjoy the coolness of the evening. They sleep the same amount of time overall, but they break up the sleep in their particular way.

Once people in our culture reach sixty or so and retire from work, they tend to start taking naps after lunch as well. Sometimes daytime napping develops out of boredom with a less active life-style. But sometimes it is simply a spontaneous indulgence of anyone who doesn't have to head back to work after lunch.

A problem with napping arises only when a person also tries to sleep the usual length of time at night. If you are sleeping in the afternoon, you will need to sleep less in the night, if you don't want to wake up groggy the next morning. More importantly, if you sleep in the afternoon, chances are you will have trouble falling asleep early in the evening, or you will wake up early in the morning because you have already had as much sleep as you need.

Again, elderly people often become frustrated and worried when they find their nighttime sleep cycles changing, and will lie awake struggling to force themselves back to sleep even though they have already had enough sleep for the night. This is a problem of habit and expectation, not of sleep itself. If you are caught up in this pattern, I advise you to either forgo the afternoon nap, or to open yourself to the magic of the early morning. Or simply change your schedule for when you go to bed, and stay up later before hitting the sack.

I say this knowing that many of you are in fact avoiding waking up at night because you have an old, negative fear of the night. Don't be embarrassed if this is the case. All of us carry into adulthood our childhood fears and attitudes, and it is only through conscious acceptance of these reactions, and regular confrontation with them, that we can move through them.

If you simply don't like the night and want to avoid it through sleep, you will probably have to deal in a positive way with this reaction as you grow older, or suffer inordinately if you continue to reject the night through sleeping pills and such. The real terror of the night is in fact the comatose state of sleeping pills, in my opinion. It is better to open yourself to the magic of darkness than to condemn yourself to the deathly blackout of drugs, don't you think?

I want to end this chapter with a spiritual meditation on darkness itself, to see if this might help you to be more open to the nighttime experiences which await you. Most of us still carry residues of the old superstitious heritage which taught us that darkness is somehow evil, sinful, of the devil himself, while light is associated with God, goodness, and all things positive. With such programming, it is no wonder that we tend to fear the night, and choose to sleep through it rather than to be awake before the dawn. Nighttime is also when the old-time predators of human beings could sneak up and grab us, because in the night we can't see what is happening around us. So it is natural to want to lock ourselves up and sleep through the night, and to come out into a new day when the sun comes up, and not before.

Put simply, we are afraid of what we cannot see. Almost all children are thus afraid of the night. They project their horrible fantasies into the darkness, and scare themselves in the process. And when they grow up, they still carry with them a negative association of the night, and of being awake when it is dark.

My challenge to you is to begin to reverse this programming, to begin to establish a better relationship with the night. Darkness is half of life, after all. It is the more mysterious half, and as we mature into adults, we are able to open ourselves more and more to this mysterious dimension of the night. Instead of running away from darkness, we can discover new, unexplored parts of ourselves through being awake sometimes at night, especially after midnight, when the full impact of the night is felt.

Let me teach you a basic meditation on the night, which might help to open up some beautiful expansive experiences as you find yourself awake late at night or early in the morning. You can tap into the special spiritual energies of that period of the night/day, and come to know what I consider to be a very important quality of consciousness which seems to be induced by such early morning reveries.

Early-Morning Meditation

1. It is best to sit upright for this meditation, so that you break free of the sleep-oriented state of mind you feel when you are lying down. Make yourself comfortable, perhaps with a blanket around you for warmth, and if it feels good, sit with your spine upright.

2. Tune into your breathing for a few moments, as you have learned already, noticing the sensation of air coming and going through your nose, and the movements in your body caused by your relaxed breathing.

3. Then expand your awareness to include your heartbeat, or your pulse somewhere in your body. Experience your breathing and your heartbeat together. This expansion of consciousness in itself is a remarkable feeling, as your whole

body suddenly becomes highly sensitive, self-aware, calmly centered in the middle of your breathing experience.

4. Now expand your awareness to include the air around you in the room, so that you feel an intimate connection between the air around you and the air you are breathing into your lungs and body. With every breath, simply allow yourself to become more and more conscious of this oneness of the outside world with your inside world.

5. Expand your awareness another step to look around you at what you see, as you absorb the impressions of the outside world and take it deep within your mind. Notice how your perception of an object changes from how you see it when you are inhaling to when you are exhaling. In this way, you can integrate your breathing and your seeing, and come to a very fine spiritual experience.

6. Also open yourself while you breathe to the sounds around you, so that you take in auditory impressions in the same way you are taking in visual impressions. Let your senses come alive in the present moment.

7. And while in this expanded level of consciousness, you can close your eyes if you want to, and open yourself to whatever deep experiences come to you. Every time you do this early-morning meditation, you will find yourself having quite a new experience, since the present moment is always new.

As an optimum daily routine, you can do this meditation at some point during the daylight hours and also do it at some point if you wake up at night, so that you have the balance of the two different experiences. The meditation is of course a basic spiritual meditation to be used as often as you choose, for generating an ongoing sense of calm and peace inside you—the exact qualities of consciousness which you need to encourage in order to move beyond insomnia.

Give it a try now if you want to. Pause, read through the description of the meditation again, and give yourself the pleasure of such an experience.

CHAPTER SEVEN

Sexual Dimensions of Sleep

There are two dimensions to consider in the relationship between sexuality and sleeping. The most obvious one has to do with the release of sexual pressures through intercourse and masturbation. People who are sexually frustrated for one reason or another do tend to have a hard time falling asleep. There is a tension in their body which directly thwarts the relaxation needed for sleep to come.

It is quite commonly known among therapists that many people living alone without a sexual partner use regular masturbation in the evening to help generate relaxation and sleep. Compared with using sleeping pills for the same purpose, this is generally considered a positive means toward an end.

The final result of masturbation is not just sexual release, but also a feeling of general well-being. This happens for two reasons. First of all, when a person masturbates, fantasies of intimacy are almost always used to induce genital stimulation. These fantasies of togetherness, usually conjured up from memories of past relationships, leave the person with that good old-time feeling of intimacy which encourages sleep.

In general, making love stimulates a feeling of oneness, of ego loss. And this feeling of letting go of one's tight ego boundaries is what must happen to us all, if we are to fall asleep. Also during lovemaking there comes a point where thoughts about the past and future are erased, so that present-moment sensations and emotions become one's entire reality. Again, when we fall asleep, this is what happens to us.

It is curious that when we talk about sleeping with someone, this can mean either that we have sexual intercourse with this person or that we go to bed and sleep beside each other without any sexual interaction at all. And of course, often we do both in the same night. There is no better sleep than that which comes after making love, as you drift off to sleep in each other's arms.

If we step back as we consider two adults in each other's loving arms, we can see quite directly that our hunger for physical intimacy comes not only from our biological urges, but also from our early experiences when we were intimate with our mothers and fathers, being held with tender acceptance and love during our early formative years.

So to sleep with someone, to be hugged and loved, touched and kissed, awakens in adults the old-time sense of security and well-being which helped us let go and drift off into sleep as children.

It is no surprise that so many cases of insomnia result from the loss of a relationship which provided this nightly sense of caring and togetherness. In fact, it is to be expected that when a person's sexual partner is missing for one reason or another, there will be at least a few nights of disturbed sleep.

Often two people who love each other very much and who feel quite secure in their relationship must spend some nights apart. Even when the security remains constant, there can be insomnia problems during the separation, problems which instantly go away with the reunion of the sleeping partners.

But when there is conflict between two lovers, or husband and wife, and they separate—even if they just sleep in different rooms—sleep disturbances are almost certain to develop. When this physical separation is compounded with the emotional anxiety of permanent separation and the loss of intimacy, then we have a condition which can predictably lead to insomnia.

Many people will resolve this condition by holding on to old fantasies of their intimacy with their loved one, even when this person is estranged from them. They will create fantasies about reunion, or lie in bed and indulge in memories about the good old times, and this will help create the relaxation and sense of togetherness needed for sleep to come. Masturbation in this situation will of course help as well.

But for a successful resolution of the separation conflict, it will be necessary to face the reality of the loss and resultant painful emotions, and to recover from the separation by regaining one's own individual center. It will probably be necessary to go through some sleepless nights of anger and loneliness, to fully experience the reality of being alone in the world. Only then, when these emotions are felt honestly and in depth, can the separation be accepted. And only at this point can one reclaim his or her separate identity, and move forward to a new relationship.

The difference between a healthy grief experience and an unhealthy one lies in whether the pain of the recovery process is surrendered to, or whether the person blocks the grief process and remains caught in the anxiety and anger of rejection over a longer period of time. This difference is usually determined by the level of maturity of the person. All of us grow up physically, but many of us remain caught in childhood emotions throughout our lives. Specifically, many of us go through adult life relating with people in the same way we related with our parents—in a dependent pattern. We are afraid to lose the love of our adult relationships, and so we play the dependent child in these relationships, attaching to a sexual mate, for instance, with the same emotional bonding that we had with our mother or father.

With such a childish emotional relationship, we are not able to act independently in life. Instead of finding our own separate center within our own selves, we continue to place our sense of security on the shoulders of our loved one. This can function throughout a relationship's life without trauma, if both parties of the relationship are satisfied with the dominant-submissive situation.

But as soon as separation occurs, disaster hits for the dependent member of the relationship. This is what so often happens to older couples when one of them dies: the surviving partner loses sleep because of suddenly having to sleep alone.

I am not, by the way, advocating that all of us learn how

to live completely independently, not needing anyone to live with and love. There is always a certain amount of mutual dependency in a deep relationship. But there is also the need for independence in a relationship, so that both partners can continue to evolve in their own centers, while sharing their lives.

If such mature individuality is nurtured in a relationship, then the trauma of separation in divorce or death can be moved through successfully. If the dependent qualities of a personality are dominant, however, the struggle to recover from the loss of a loved one, or even the loss of a long-term job, can prove extremely difficult. It is in this situation that many people become addicted to sleeping pills and mood elevators. They are in need of a dependency of some sort, and if there is no new person upon whom to become dependent, then the drugs will be seen as better than nothing.

From the outside, it is easy for me to sit here and outline the psychological dimensions of dependency and the traumas of separation. But I know that from the inside, such explanations can hardly help to relieve the symptoms of sleepless nights and addictive habits. What is needed are some realistic pathways one can follow to begin to break out of dependency relationships and to recover from depression and the sense of isolation that loss of a loved one can cause.

The most important path which I am offering in this book is that of honest reflection on your present life, and particular meditations which you can do regularly to stimulate the finding of your own independent center. The first step in such growth is always to look at your thoughts and feelings honestly, to see yourself just as you are, and to accept yourself. If you are strung out on sleeping pills and uppers and living a solitary life that makes you want to cry out in anguish, then your first step is to admit to this situation rather than trying to hide your actual condition from yourself and others.

The first step toward improving a life condition is that step of learning to observe one's day-to-day thoughts, so that you can see how your thoughts are constantly holding you in that very state of mind and emotion from which you are suffering and want to escape.

Perhaps the bottom-line realization which stimulates a

release from insomnia is this: there is no getting away from yourself. No amount of thinking, no amount of problem-solving, no amount of drugs, no amount of socializing or money-making will ever move you even one iota away from yourself. So no matter how terrible you think you are, you are stuck with yourself. Your past happened just as it did. And if you can't come to see yourself clearly and accept yourself despite all your imperfections, then you face a lifetime of drugs and mind-games and other unsuccessful attempts to escape from yourself.

I am speaking strongly and bluntly in this chapter because I know you are opening your heart to helping yourself, or you would not have read this far in a book such as this. You have already turned your personal corner and are headed in a positive direction. Now what you need are tools to work with, a few of which I have offered you already. If you find at some point that you need some professional help as well, I hope that you can reach out confidently, knowing that the very act of reaching out for help is an act of independence. (You might also read my book *Finding Each Other* for special guidance in interpersonal growth.)

To round out this chapter, I want to offer you a process for clarifying your intimate needs, so that if in fact you are suffering from a loss of human contact and intimacy, you can see clearly what you need to strive for, in order to reestablish a new sense of sexual intimacy and belonging.

Clarifying Your Intimate Needs

If you are having difficulties in falling asleep, take an honest look at your present intimate situation. What or who do you need to come into your life so that you can again relax, feel good in your heart and body, and surrender to a deep sleep?

It is usually best to assume that bygones are bygones, and not to dwell on the possibility of getting back into an old relationship that has hit the rocks. The same is true about an old job you lost, or any other situation that used to give you that sense of security which enabled you to sleep at night.

Instead, begin to open yourself for a movement into a new relationship which will bring you the satisfaction and security you need. Take time now, and during the next few days, to reflect deeply on what needs you have that are not being satisfied, and how you can act to find someone to satisfy them. Are you able to grow and come to a deeper feeling of independence so that you do not need someone in your life who provides the security you hunger for—or are you in fact someone who does need an intimate partner to live with, to give you the comfort that leads to good sleep? Be as honest as you can, stay aware of your breaths while your feelings rise up, and see what insights come to you.

CHAPTER EIGHT

Break the Worry Habit

When we find ourselves unable to sleep, there are almost always particular emotions which hold us in their grip and which perpetuate our sleepless condition. In order to move beyond sleepless nights, it is important to identify these "insomnia emotions" and learn how to transcend them.

Let me list the seven primary culprits and then say a brief word about each of them. Then in this chapter we will explore in depth the last three on the list, leaving the first four for later chapters. As you read the list, see which ones strike you as your main sleepless companions: frustration . . . anger . . . hopelessness . . . depression . . . worrying . . . anxiety . . . panic . . .

Frustration and *anger* are caused both by the immediate situation in which you want to get to sleep but cannot, and also by pent-up emotions which are insisting on release. Many people suffering from insomnia are in fact of the personality type which has great difficulty in expressing anger during the day—so at night these feelings come back to haunt them. Only by honestly expressing your anger can you move beyond it.

Hopelessness can also be both immediate and long-term in its source. Insomnia does put you in a situation where you know you must get to sleep in order to be ready for the next day, but in fact you absolutely cannot get to sleep. This is a hopeless position to find yourself in. However, often insomnia is just another manifestation of a person's basic attitude toward life as a hopeless experience. People who are still caught up in dependency relationships are especially prone to have this attitude, since they are prisoners in relationships that they fear to break out of.

The next common insomniac emotion is that terrible condition which is experienced in epidemic proportions: *depression.* Many doctors and psychiatrists consider depression to be the number-one cause of insomnia. Curiously enough, depression is not really an emotion at all. It is a blocked state of another emotion: anger. In the following chapter we will take a look at techniques to break free of the trait that causes such powerful suppression of any direct expression of this powerful emotion.

In this chapter we are going to focus specifically on the final three emotions on our list: *worrying, anxiety,* and *panic,* all of which emerge from the root emotion of fear. When we are afraid for any reason at all, sleep simply does not come. So we need to take a bold look at the sources of the types of fear that plague insomnia victims, and explore ways of overcoming these habitual traumas.

First, let's consider what seems to be the most innocent cause of insomnia: that of not being able to fall asleep because you are worrying about some particular situation that you will be confronting the next day. Businesspersons are famous for this habitual problem-solving mental activity in the middle of almost every night. And they insist that there is no emotional dimension to their insomnia at all. They simply cannot turn off their work-minds when there is a problem facing them that needs resolution.

These people often spend almost all of their waking lives caught up in problem-solving mind-states. They are addicts to this survival-of-the-fittest mental condition. Their prime satisfaction in life is striving to gain dominance and success in the tough competitive world they live in. Their condition seems to be the opposite of a dependent personality—they are the epitome of the rugged individualist struggling to make it on his or her own against overwhelming odds.

When these businessmen and women finally break down from the stress of their days and nights, they come dragging into my office in serious confusion and apprehension. Usually only at that unfortunate point of deterioration do they finally begin the ultimate challenge of a businessperson—that of looking honestly at their manic, compulsive survival habits, to see how they managed to sacrifice all the genuine pleasures and satisfactions of human life in their crazy push for power and piles of money.

If you are one of these tough executives who suffer from not being able to turn off your competitive, problem-solving mind at night, you should find the programs in this book relatively easy to succeed with—but you will have to understand that success in getting to sleep means letting go of worldly concerns while you sleep. This is your big challenge: letting go.

What is this drive for success anyway? Why does it get out of control and dominate a person's life so destructively? Obvious to an outside observer but not at all obvious to someone caught up in the rat race is that the men and women on the business battlefield are constantly creating life-or-death emotional situations in their lives. As far as they are concerned, with each battle for success and dominance in the business world they are right on the edge of survival itself.

When a person is constantly caught up in the struggle for survival, there is created in that person habitual stress, and this stress comes ultimately from the fear of losing the battle and, on psychological levels at least, facing death itself. The manic energy that pushes businesspeople into breakdowns and heart attacks is stimulated by this fear of not making it, of losing the battle for survival.

And it is this hidden but acute anxiety that underlies the nightly problem-solving bouts of insomnia, during which the businessperson simply cannot relax, cannot turn off the mind which is struggling with strategies of attack and victory in the next day's battlefield.

Curiously, one of the rules of Samurai warriors is that you must know how to turn off your warrior-mind each night so that you get enough sleep—otherwise you will surely lose the battle the next morning. But our contemporary business warriors are unfortunately not trained in many of the fine arts of traditional warriors, and thus they are suffering regularly both from insomnia at night and failures the next day.

What can you do to turn off your problem-solving mind? What can you do to stop the flow of thoughts which are stimulating a constant adrenaline rush in your body, which then stimulates more anxiety and frustration and intensifies the problem-solving mind-set as you fixate on future battles rather than tuning into your need for physical and mental rest and restoration?

First of all, you must recognize what you are doing to yourself through such mental behavior. In your compulsive pushing to make more money and keep the financial bogeyman from your door, you are killing yourself just as surely as if you were forcing yourself to into battle with no sleep the night before.

Sometimes businesspeople have to get knocked down with a heart attack before they can see what they have made of their lives. But hopefully if you are in this insomnia syndrome you can use the symptom of sleeplessness as your stimulus for transforming your life-style.

Bedtime is rest-time. You must make an agreement with your competitive self that gives equal value to your physical health and emotional sanity—and not take your problems to bed with you. When you lie down in bed, promise yourself that you won't think about work. And if you start thinking compulsively about what you are going to do the next day or week or year, immediately get up from bed and go into another room.

This is a basic technique which I want to teach all of you who have insomnia: you need to make your bedroom a special place where you do nothing but relax and sleep a good night's sleep. I'm going to devote an entire chapter later on to this theme of magical bedtime rituals, since they are so vital to breaking free of insomnia habits.

Another prime technique for businesspeople (and anyone who is continually caught up in problem-solving thought patterns at night) is the meditation I taught you already for relaxing your mind and moving into a direct sensory encounter with the present moment. Do you remember the process? Breath awareness/jaw relaxation/pelvic movement/toes and fingers/whole-body stretch/yawn/total relaxation.

If you will commit yourself to doing this meditation after you get into bed, you will be well on your way toward breaking free of chronic thinking-thinking-thinking (worrying-worrying-worrying) when you are trying to fall asleep. It is a highly effective process which you can tap into if you want to genuinely help yourself.

Another technique for breaking free of worrying about the future is to consider what will happen if you fail at what you are doing. It is amazing that businesspeople worth several hundred thousand dollars will treat a ten-thousand-dollar deal as if it were a life-or-death situation. They have lost a vital perspective on their lives, and are chronically behaving as if every little battle threatens their very existence.

To begin to recognize this habit—overstimulation resulting from doubts about one's survival—is to make a great step away from compulsive nighttime worrying and planning for the future. Jesus gave the perfect bedtime meditation for this with his "Consider the lilies" reflection. Do human beings really have to live in chronic stress in order to survive, or is there a more advanced level of survival in which rest and relaxation are equally valued and respected, and regularly tuned into?

Let's expand our discussion of worrying another notch now, to include all of you who chronically find yourselves lying in bed at night with your heads buzzing with future plans, hopes, uncertainties, anxieties, etc. What are you doing to yourself, and how can you break out of the habits that seem to victimize you night after night?

First of all, let's examine the basic pattern that creates a sleepless night. You get into bed, and as soon as you hit the pillow, your mind starts thinking about the coming day, about the challenges that face you which need preparation. And before you even see it coming, your mind has slammed itself into the full-steam-ahead gear of problem-solving activity.

Such problem-solving mental behavior is based on fantasy, right? You must imagine something that might happen in the future, and then play out different fantasy versions of what could develop, based on different strategies you might take. Should you do this or that tomorrow? What game plan will bring victory?

And while you are imagining all this, you are also stimulating the emotions which would accompany success or failure. Your muscles actually respond to the activities you are imagining, so that tensions develop throughout your body. Furthermore, the emotions which you are stimulating through your thoughts will directly result in glandular secretions that put adrenaline in your bloodstream—and there you are, tense, excited, and agitated, and absolutely unable to sleep a wink for hours on end.

Thinking about the future ruins your chances of getting rested in preparation for the future. It is really extremely foolish to indulge in such worrying and problem-solving, when your biggest problem to be solved is how to get to sleep in the present moment.

You see, when you take your mental attention away from the present moment and put it into the future, as you always do in the process of worrying and problem-solving, you are in essence deserting your body, which exists only here in the present moment. This is the great problem with thinking in general—you go into remembering the past, or imagining a possible future, and lose the present moment.

Sleep, however, happens only right here, right now. If you want your body to drift into sleep, you must turn your attention to sensory experiences rather than to thoughts. This is such a basic fact, but one which we so often overlook.

Ultimately, what good does all your worrying do anyway? You are going to die sometime, you are not going to succeed in problem-solving your way out of your mortality. And in the meantime, instead of lying there in painful tense anticipation of what might come in the future, why don't you just tune into your body in the present moment and give yourself the chance to feel good right now?

Sleep comes when you make this step. We tend to fall asleep when we feel good, not when we feel tense. So what is your relationship with feeling good? Why are you chronically torturing yourself with habitual worrying about the future? What does your common sense tell you to do?

It is often said in professional circles that insomnia is nothing more than a bad case of free-floating anxiety. This is certainly true of the kind of insomnia we are talking about in this chapter. And this condition of free-floating anxiety is so dominant in our culture these days that it has almost become the norm. It seems natural for us to be worrying about what is going to happen in the world, for instance.

We sit in front of our television sets night after night, taking in all the atrocious events discussed on the nightly news, and then we expect ourselves to be able to sleep after seeing the very worst things we could imagine, in living color on the boob tube. No wonder we are anxious, when we constantly bombard our minds and emotions with the horrors of the world.

If you are someone who worries too much, sell your television! Stop reading the newspapers. Throw away your weekly newsmagazines. If the world is going to blow up tomorrow, are you really any better off for having worried yourself sick for years in advance about the possibility?

One of my conditions for working with clients who suffer from insomnia is that they stop watching television, and that they stop reading the news media's publications for a month. I know that this sounds like very severe deprivation to force on someone in the modern world. But I hate to waste my time working with a client who is then going directly home and taking in media poisons which stimulate the very conditions we are working to eliminate—anxiety and sleeplessness, and all the problems which result from them.

So I suggest to you, without being so strict as I am with my clients, that you avoid news sources which make you worry about the world situation. I assure you that you can survive quite happily without the news media's constant barrage of disasters. You can ask a friend to give you a phone call if something is mentioned in the news that you should know about for your personal life. But how often does the news offer such worthwhile information?

Otherwise, just let go of being plugged into that dimension of the world. Who needs it really? The news media play on our sense of insecurity, they hook us on their shows because it is human nature to want to know if something terrible is happening in the world. See if you can break your TV addiction and stop programming your mind with anxiety-provoking news shows.

When you watch the evening news your body reacts to what you see, and tensions spread throughout your system. Then you go to bed with your head full of maimed bodies and nuclear holocaust and economic disaster and so on and so forth—and do you really expect to be able to sleep with this in your mind? And if you do sleep, what kind of dreams do you expect to have?

Perhaps the worst thing that has happened to older citizens in our culture in the last fifty years is the advent of television. It keeps you company if you are alone, and entertains you when you are too old to get out and entertain yourself—but look at the damage it wreaks on your system. You experience paranoia as a habitual emotional state because of all the violence you see on television. You feel depressed because you see the hopeless condition of the world day after day all around the globe. And you feel isolated and terribly alone when you watch the schmaltzy idealized family dramas that are shown on television.

What is worse is this: rather than getting out and making real live human contact with people around you, you sit there alone with artificial social stimulation gained through the bombardment of television energy. With all your neighbors likewise glued to the tube, there is actually no one out there to make contact with in terms of genuine human touching and social intercourse.

So please don't think me so stringent or fanatic when I say throw your television away if you want to get over insomnia. TV is not a natural stimulation, it is an agitation to the system, and thus an enemy to peace, to sensory pleasure, to human relating and certainly to deep peaceful sleep at night.

As a final note, consider again the tribal story of the group out in the Kalahari desert. They had no television. They were terribly poor. Business success was something unknown to them. They were without money. They even had to sleep outside where very real dangers surrounded them. But they slept a good night's sleep, and they laughed a great deal every day, and the old folks were an amazement to me, so vital with life even as they were heading off to the great oasis in the sky in the near future.

If you suffer from the plague of free-floating anxiety which keeps you awake at night, I want to say this: it isn't just your problem, and you aren't personally to blame. We are caught up in a vast sociological condition in which all of us feel this general underlying anxiety about life. So instead of thinking that there is something wrong just with you, hold in mind that there is something wrong with the way we as an entire culture are handling our emotional responses to being alive on this planet. We are chronically overstimulating ourselves with thoughts and media impressions which create anxiety in our systems. This is actually quite a crazy thing to do to ourselves.

What can you do about it? You can definitely take your own life-style in your own hands, and let it begin to evolve consciously in healthy, enjoyable directions. Instead of spending hours a day watching television, you can spend hours a day making your little corner of the world a better place to live in. And by thus increasing your own good feelings, you increase the good feelings of the whole world. If all of us were to do this positive act of spreading heartfelt joy, rather than absorbing anxiety and depression, what a better world it would be!

The Good News Meditation

With this in mind, let's end this chapter with a simple meditation you can do many times a day to directly augment the good feelings of the present moment while turning off the worrying thought patterns which might otherwise continue to ruin your days and nights. Again, the trick is to turn your attention to the present moment, which is the only place you are going to find genuine satisfying pleasure and relaxation in life—this is the good news, that the present moment is still here, and we can instantly tap into it.

The meditation goes as follows, and you can either memorize it so you can do it regularly without effort, or take advantage of the guided cassette sessions which lead you through the meditation.

You turn your attention to your breathing as you have learned to do in previous exercises, feeling the air coming and going through your nose and the movements in your chest and belly as you breathe . . . and even if you are in pain somewhere in your body, you now turn your attention to a place in your body where you find good feelings. Just let your breathing continue as your primary focus, while you open yourself to exploring every part of your body, until you

ind a region that feels good. Perhaps you will want to move
a little, to generate the good feeling, since movement often
does feel good. . . . Allow your mind to be filled with the
present moment, with your breathing, and also with good
feelings you locate in your body. . . . You can do this with
eyes closed, or with eyes open and looking at something in
your room that is aesthetically beautiful to behold, so that
you fill your visual realms with beauty as well . . . and as
you remain in this meditative state, notice how your
breathing relaxes, softens, becomes more regular and deep,
bringing a beautiful sense of peace which you can immerse
yourself in. . . .

CHAPTER NINE

Releasing Repressed Frustrations

To become angry when one is frustrated in one way or another is a perfectly normal and healthy human emotion. We are born with the anger response preprogrammed into our very genes. Babies cry with a vigorous show of anger when anything at all goes wrong in their daily routines. And as they get older and can walk and manifest their frustrations more physically, their crying tantrums turn into quite a violent show of physical aggression when they become enraged through frustration.

Why is it that so many grown-ups have such difficulty in expressing their frustrations directly toward the particular people who stimulate this emotion?

The answer is simple—when we are afraid of the consequences of our angry outbursts, we try to block our anger so as to avoid punishment of one sort or another.

Almost all ingrained inhibitions related to the expression of anger develop early in a person's life, when the personality is taking shape in response to parental guidance and discipline. This is certainly true with the expression or the inhibition of anger. Many parents wisely allow toddlers to express their wild aggressiveness (within reasonable limits), because it is this very expression of early self-assertion which helps create a sense of independence and self-confidence in a child. Such early freedom to test one's personal limits is the groundwork for the development of a mature, responsible personality.

But all too often, parents react to childhood anger and aggression in an overly negative, judgmental way. They see such infantile expressions of physical violence as somehow wrong, usually in the framework of a religious belief system. And by making the unfortunate error of equating childish expressions of violence with later adult expressions of the same emotion, they restrict the freedom of the child to push and struggle against authority.

Children who are severely punished for expressing their frustrations, especially those who have parental love withdrawn when they become angry and self-willed, will usually grow up with underdeveloped wills, with weak egos, with overly dependent and childish ways of relating with people around them.

In a word, they will be afraid to express their feelings, believing that their feelings would create conflict and possible separation between themselves and their important relationships. When they feel the urge to break free and act on their own in a relationship, an old inhibition will grab at them with anxiety and block the independent action—this is the nature of a dependent personality.

But with every inhibition of an independent action or thought, the dependent person also feels a frustration at being held somehow prisoner in the relationship. Anger which has been held inside since early childhood rises up to the surface with every little suppression of feeling—and this buried anger, this repressed expression of will, is constantly disturbing this person's sleeping and waking consciousness.

Often with clients I have worked with, there existed a mother or father who for various ego reasons needed the child to be overly dependent on them. This neurotic attachment to the child expressed itself through not letting the child feel separate and independent from the parent. Instead, the child grew up without having adequate experiences of personal power and freedom—and remained under the illusion that he or she could not really survive without the constant support, love, acceptance, and advice of the parent.

All of us, of course, were once dependent on our parents. Life is a progression from total dependence to more or less successful independence—from childhood to mature adulthood. The trauma of breaking free of the parental world is something we all have to face at some point in our lives. And in fact none of us completely breaks free of being dependent on others for our survival. Life is a balance between mutual interdependence and independent action.

In terms of insomnia, the evidence from many different sources seems quite conclusive that the more emotionally dependent a person remains in adulthood, the more severe the reaction will be to any separation from a loved one.

Furthermore, unless this underlying quality of dependence and emotional immaturity is faced and let go of, the same old insomnia patterns will recur each time any kind of separation from a primary relationship occurs, or is even vaguely hinted at.

I mentioned just in passing in the last chapter that when anger is denied expression as a regular habit, the resulting development in a personality is depression. This is why people with depressive conditions so often suffer from insomnia. They suppress their entire functioning in life in an unconscious effort to block any flooding of powerful angry energy through their systems. Only when they lie down and try to go to sleep does this buried anger have a chance to break through the habits of inhibition and express itself. With such an upsurge of emotional turmoil coming every time a depressed person moves toward sleep, it is no wonder that sleep is impossible.

If you often find yourself caught up in aggressive, angry thoughts and emotions when you are trying to get to sleep, what can you do to overcome this habit?

Of course, here is where most people jump toward the open hand offering a sleeping pill. It is important to understand that both depressive mind-states and the effects induced by sleeping pills serve the same supposedly beneficial purpose of inhibiting the forbidden feelings of anger and aggression in a person. If you are deathly afraid of what might happen if you blew your top and released all your buried emotions toward your marital partner or your boss or anyone with whom you are afraid to be emotionally honest— then any trick that blocks this dangerous emotion will be welcomed into your life-style, even if you suffer considerably from this trick, as does anyone with a depressive condition or a drug habit.

My main training in my early days as a therapist was in the bioenergetic tradition, where we were champions in helping clients to make contact with, and triumphantly release, their blocked charges of anger and aggression. There is a great wisdom in this therapeutic tradition of Wilhelm Reich and his many followers, and I still consider it a blessing for anyone who is thus blocked, if they can afford and are able to find a good emotional-release therapist to work with. It is a tremendous healing experience even for those of you who consider yourselves quite healthy emotionally. There's always room to grow.

But it is important to keep in mind when you are seeking to break free of your inhibitions and express your anger directly that between you and this expression is a lot of fear and trembling. Early-childhood anxieties related to expressing forbidden emotions run extremely deep and powerful. And you will want to do some serious reflection on the fears which underlie your inhibitions, in order to succeed in opening yourself up to positive growth and maturation.

Consider the following description of an all-too-common life situation: you are in a relationship with a person (or a job) which you constantly fear losing. You become anxious at the very thought of losing your loved one whom you need so very much. And because of this fear of being alone in life, you are afraid to do anything or to say anything that might threaten your relationship.

Therefore, you live your life in a restricted manner, feeling confined, unable to really step out and do your own thing in life. Even when you feel the urge to do something risky which would satisfy a deep need in you, something blocks your spontaneous action and holds you back. Your voice tends to be high and whiny, and you are a habitual complainer about the condition of the world. You find fault with everything around you in a subtle way. You are an excellent critic because of this frustration with how other people behave and live their lives.

You also complain that people don't care enough for you, and you find yourself all too often fuming inside because of the shortcomings of others in their concern for you. Sometimes you are manic and so speedy that you can hardly sit on your energy charge, while other times you are empty of energy, down in the dumps, depressed about everything around you.

In either case you often find your emotions in a turmoil, and especially when it comes time to sleep, every little thing bothers you. Sleep eludes you. Anxieties torment you and you attach your anxieties onto anything you can find in your environment, even if you know deep down that you aren't being fair sometimes to the people around you. You feel an enduring sense of frustration in life, both in how your days go and how your nights go as well. Something is wrong, but you can't put your finger on anything that helps your condition.

Often you go around acting like you are happy and positive, smiling until it hurts. But underneath your superficial brightness there is a depression which makes everything seem vaguely unreal and definitely unfulfilling.

Quite naturally the person on whom you depend for your sense of emotional survival has a somewhat difficult time relating with you day in and day out. Because you need this person desperately, but resent this person's unconscious control over your life, there are consistent tensions between you. And these tensions naturally make you feel insecure—exactly the feeling that creates sleepless nights.

What a syndrome!

Beyond Dependency

If this general life-sketch rings bells, how can you act as a conscious adult right now and in the coming days and weeks and months, to begin to evolve into a more independent, less anxious, more assertive person?

1. First of all, regularly look back into your past. Begin to develop a more pragmatic understanding of your relationship with your mother and your father. To what extent did they let you develop your own sense of self, as opposed to keeping you dependent on them emotionally? And what habits did you develop as a child with your parents which you are perpetuating now in your present relationship?

Just that paragraph alone might take you months to explore. I am throwing out to you quite major keys in rapid succession here—so I hope you will read through this list of suggestions and then go back and consider each one at more length.

2. A second suggestion for developing a more expansive, independent life-style is this: begin to notice how many of your personal decisions you let your partner make for you, as if you were still a child letting your parents make all your decisions for you. Each time you play out this dependent role in your present life, notice it! And begin to see times when you can act on your own—seek out these opportunities, in fact.

3. Begin as well to take conscious note of your independent accomplishments in life. Often dependent people completely ignore and cast away the ego pleasures of doing something on their own. If you do this self-negation routine, begin to notice the habit, and consciously look at your daily life with an eye to recognizing your achievements. This is an extremely important ego-building process. Every day, keep a diary that lists what independent decisions and accomplishments you made!

4. Also, jump into the question of what underlies your regular sense of frustration and anger at the world. See beyond your critical thought patterns and accept that underneath your criticism of the world around you is a sense of your own lack of self-worth. Is this true for you?

If so, your challenge is to begin to build up your own relationship with yourself. Respect is the key word here. Demand respect from others for what you accomplish, and give it to yourself as well.

5. And especially, begin to look into the giant realm called conflict. The majority of the people I work with who suffer from disturbed sleep are people who have extreme difficulty dealing with conflict situations. They avoid them like the plague, with an abnormal anxiety associated with any confrontation related to important relationships in their lives.

Thus when they would normally need to stand their ground and disagree with someone, they block the assertive feelings welling up in them, and back down in the confrontation. They let other people walk all over them because they offer no resistance; and then they fume secretly about these people's lack of concern and respect.

If you tend to do this, then the time has come to begin to learn to hold your ground in life, to insist openly on what you think is right. Otherwise, you're going to toss and turn in bed for the rest of your life, creating angry fantasy scenes of expressing your assertive impulses—instead of releasing this energy in the appropriate place at the time the confrontation actually happened.

I know that I am telling you to jump into the fire and work through patterns of behavior that are very deeply ingrained in your personality. But what else can I do, and what else can *you* do if you really want to break free of your nightly bouts of insomnia? Do what you can for yourself, with the tools I am offering. Get hold of books that more specifically apply to some of these themes which I have just mentioned, if you feel the need for more guidance of this sort. And also reach out to your community for help. If you are of a religious persuasion, assert yourself by walking into your minister's office and tell him or her that you are struggling with the challenge of becoming more assertive in life. See what resources he or she can suggest. And look elsewhere as well. Workshops have become almost a cliché, but many of them are still dynamite opportunities to get in a group situation and express yourself in new ways. We grow both through inner reflection and through external, social expression and risk-taking. You can balance both in a positive game plan for moving beyond old inhibitions.

6. Every breath you breathe is actually an assertion of your independent status on this planet. You don't have to look for exotic experiences to begin to recreate your sense of self-worth and freedom. Just turn your attention to the air you are breathing right now. You are free to breathe it in any way you want to, correct?

You can breathe the air with shallow tight inhales and barely visible exhales, as one does when afraid—or you can change your breathing consciously, step by step, so that you are breathing with more power, with more confidence, and with more pleasure as well. The way you breathe is who you are. And because your breathing is under your conscious control—when you take such control—you are right now in position to alter your stance in the world.

First of all, simply notice honestly how you are now breathing. What emotion is expressed by the way you are breathing? This emotion, right now, is you. There is no separation between how you are breathing and who you are. And your breathing doesn't lie. It is a barometer of your deepest feelings.

It is also the kingpin that determines if and when you fall asleep at night. Unless you are breathing in a relaxed way, you simply cannot fall asleep. This is basic reality. The way you breathe is one and the same with the emotion you are feeling. And the emotion you are feeling determines whether you sleep or don't sleep. To lie in bed and reflect on this primal fact is one of the finest meditations which can move you effortlessly toward sleep.

So—I have taken a general shot in your direction with this chapter and its suggestions. Naturally some of what I said might not apply to you at all, but perhaps some of it does. The challenge for you now is to take what made sense and act upon it.

Emotional Balancing and Release Techniques

There are times, when you lie in bed with your body a tense knot of muscles and nerves, when it would be helpful to directly encourage the flow of pent-up emotions up and out your mouth—to discharge your feelings so that your muscles can relax and your mind be free. Let me give you a brief outline of two particular techniques which just might be crucial in your quest for successful ways to break through tensions and fall asleep. If you find that your emotions are so blocked or so explosive that you cannot do these techniques just from the book, you can also use the supplementary guided sessions or seek out professional guidance. But for most of you, knowing a structured process should be all you need for opening yourself to emotional release and balancing.

Emotional Release

The first key to emotional release is the conscious act of breathing through the mouth, so that your main vehicle for expressing your feelings—your voice—is free to sound off. People who toss and turn all night almost always do so with tense jaw muscles and a closed mouth. This chronic bodily stance makes emotional release quite impossible. Thus the extreme frustration felt in the body.

So whenever you are caught in the throes of insomnia, practice the "open mouth" meditation—breathe and let some sounds come out, so that your anger and frustration, your hopelessness and fears can start to find release.

The other variable of emotional release is your whole body, which carries tension whenever an emotion is blocked from expression. This tension directly inhibits the sleep response, as we have already seen.

Try this: lie on your back in bed, and as you breathe through the mouth, pound your arms on the bed on either side of you, and kick with your feet too. Make these movements of aggression, like a little child kicking and shouting in a temper tantrum. See how far you can go into this energetic discharge of your pent-up feelings. If you can surrender to your anger and express it, blow it off, then you will almost certainly find yourself much more ready to go to sleep after the discharge.

And very often, after you release the anger inside you, you will find yourself softening and starting to cry, releasing the feelings of hopelessness and loneliness, so that you open up to a surge of expansive feelings once the tears are done.

Remember throughout to keep breathing through your mouth, so you don't shut off the flow of emotions. Your habit will almost certainly be to shut your mouth. See if you can consciously breathe through the mouth as often as possible, if you are a chronic blocker of your emotions. Let the pressure come up and out of your chest. The feeling of relief will be instant and important.

I recommend that you do some variation of the emotional release session several times a day if possible, so that by bedtime you aren't carrying a large charge of unwanted emotional pressure inside you. Of course it takes time to learn how to let go of your emotions, so you will need to discipline yourself to do this session until you reach the point where you fully surrender to it.

Balancing Your Emotions

The other technique I want to teach you is one I have been developing in my therapy practice over the years and which can be applied very effectively to insomnia conditions. What you need to do is to spend a couple of minutes indulging in one particular emotion, anger for instance. See if you can feel anger in your muscles, remember times when you were angry, and fantasize situations in which you express powerful angry feelings.

Then after you have briefly made deep contact with this emotion, let go of that emotion, and consciously start to feel an opposite emotion inside you, such as *playfulness*. For a couple of minutes, remember times when you were playing, imagine being playful, enjoying yourself without a care in your mind. By shifting from anger to playfulness as a conscious meditation, you learn how to break free of the compulsive emotional fixations which plague you in the night.

After playfulness, shift into feeling *grief and despair* for a couple of minutes, and fully indulge in these feelings, letting yourself cry if you want to, and relive times when you were overwhelmed by these feelings. Almost certainly such emotions are present in your insomnia anyway.

But here's the magic of this "emotional balancing" session—after a couple of minutes of feeling grief and hopelessness, shift out of those feelings as a conscious act of will. Discover that in fact you are not a victim of your emotions. You can use your will to turn your attention to other emotions when you want to. In this case, turn your attention to *the feeling of love*, of having your heart open to someone, and enjoying the beautiful sensation of being a loving person. Let memories come, and indulge in this part of your personality, the loving side of you, for a couple of minutes.

Then let go of that feeling, and shift your emotional attention to *repulsion*, to that feeling of not being able to stand something or someone, of feeling actually nauseous about something you are doing, or someone you are with.

Then after a couple of minutes, you can let go of this feeling, and open yourself to its opposite, to the feeling of *bliss, peace, total contentment*. Now that you have felt a mixture of feelings, you can relax and take more time to open yourself to the pure sensations which come after discharging all the various emotions. Let peace come into you as the aftermath of the emotional balancing experience. Breathe into an expansive sensation in your chest, and make yourself comfortable in bed so you can drift into sleep. . . .

I hope that you will take very seriously these two powerful techniques for freeing your body and mind of emotional tensions. If you want further explanations of the process of emotional balancing and release, you can turn to my book *Immune-System Activation,* which deals with these techniques in depth, and also use the cassette programs to guide you into the experiences I just outlined.

Right now, pause for a few breaths, breathe through your mouth, and see what emotions might want to come up and out.

CHAPTER TEN

Bedtime Rituals

Regardless of the particular origins of your bouts of insomnia, there are practical rituals you can perform each day to help you sleep better at night.

Before making those suggestions, however, I want to discuss what I mean by the word *ritual*. I don't mean any particular religious program when I speak of a ritual. Instead I am referring to the universal human habit of establishing certain regularly repeated routines in daily life—routines which in one way or another have the power to affect our thoughts, emotions, and general physiological condition.

A ritual, in other words, is a repeated movement, sound, thought, or a combination of these three elements which carries a special meaning for us because of its association with other dimensions of our life. A ritual can be as simple as a regular good-night kiss from Papa or as complex in meaning as the Holy Communion.

The key to a powerful ritual lies in its association with important aspects of our lives. Turning a light off is, in itself, an insignificant physical act of our fingers. But this action can develop strong ritualistic associations if every night for ten years this is the last act you perform before going to bed.

We are ultimately creatures of habit, and rituals are of course glorified habits which we raise to a level of special significance. If we nurture the significance of a ritual, then the ritual becomes more powerful in our lives. If we let a ritual drop down to a meaningless habit to which we pay no attention, then its power in our lives has been lost.

So in looking for ways to enhance your sleeping potential, it is very effective to consider the rituals which you perform before going to bed—and begin to give them more conscious associative powers for inducing sleep.

What do you do each night before going to bed? What are your regular habits? What is the sequence of actions which you perform during the last half hour before you finally climb into your bed?

I encourage you to take this exploration of your nighttime rituals quite seriously. In fact, it would be best if you got out paper and pen and started working out a list of everything you regularly or semi-regularly do during the half hour before getting into bed. Take enough time working on this list so that you get a complete accounting of all your nightly activities—and then work to get this list in a fairly accurate order of what you do first, second, third, etc.

For instance, most of us turn off certain lights in a certain order before going to bed. We brush our teeth and perform other bathroom rituals on a regular basis. Perhaps we look at ourselves in the mirror, put on facial cream, pee a final time, etc. What do you do? If you aren't sure, be certain to take note of what you do tonight as you actually walk through your rituals of preparation for bed.

What social interactions, if any, do you usually include in preparations for bed? If you live with other people, what good-night rituals are customary, giving you a feeling of communal togetherness as you head for bed? And if you sleep alone in your home, what thoughts go through your mind, who do you think of upon retiring to bed? These are very important rituals which almost everyone performs in one way or another—but which are often violated during periods of emotional stress and resultant insomnia.

Once in bed, what are your usual habits of behavior? Do you watch television, read, masturbate, make love, lie in bed imagining fantasy experiences, worry, problem-solve? Make a list of these habits over the next few nights, and gain a clear, conscious understanding of your nightly mental rituals and physical actions.

I want to go through a list of recommended rituals which

you might like to include in your nightly activities, rituals which have proven effective for others and should help you fall asleep as well. There are also certain common rituals which are counterproductive to a good night's sleep that I want to talk over with you.

Regular Daily Exercise

As biological organisms, we are blessed with a large daily supply of muscular energy with which to carry out our regular activities. This energy is a genetic endowment; we could call it the life-force itself. We are energetic creatures, and we must manage our energy supplies wisely or suffer from serious difficulties.

Many people who suffer from insomnia are for one reason or another not adequately burning up their daily supply of physical energy. When bedtime comes, this energy naturally generates restlessness in the body and hyperactivity in the mind. There is a frustration deep down in one's being when physical energy remains in the system.

People who are depressed during the day are especially vulnerable to this physiological dimension of insomnia, because they have been lethargic throughout the daylight hours, repressing physical movement instead of enjoying it. Such is also the case with people who are chained to a desk all day at work, and don't have much chance for physical labor or play.

If this describes you, then you should try to increase your physical activities each day. If you lie in bed tossing and turning all night, and want to do something about it, then it is essential that you discipline yourself enough to at least get up and out the next day for a good half-hour walk in the fresh air. If at all possible, run a while too. You don't have to take up serious jogging to get enough exercise. Just put on some tennis shoes when you go for a walk, and intermittently jog for a few minutes, then walk for a few minutes. Even if you are elderly and don't see yourself as a jet-set jogger, push yourself into a gear just one step faster than a brisk walk, so that you come alive with the wild primitive spirit which running magically wakes up inside you. Of course, be sure to moderate this suggestion if the condition of your health requires less strenuous exercise.

I also strongly recommend swimming whenever possible at your local pool, and of course all the other athletic activities that might be available in your neighborhood. It doesn't matter what sort of exercise you get. All that matters is that you move around vigorously for long enough to experience that essential release of your physical power!

Evening Movement Programs

Many people join evening classes in movement at their local adult education centers when insomnia is a problem. Any sort of dancing, at home or in a group, is highly recommended, as well as the classic and effective hatha yoga classes which exist in almost every community these enlightened days.

If you are going to do movement programs in the evening, *make sure that you don't exercise strenuously just before going to bed.* An hour before is fine. But just before bedtime I recommend only quiet stretching such as yoga, or perhaps gentle free-form dancing. Don't do anything that gets the heart pumping and the adrenaline flowing, or you will have to wait for this to abate before sleep will come to you.

Another wonderful form of exercise is of course making love, and many people jump into bed and use this magical God-given technique for burning away the final tensions of the day. However, when there are relationship conflicts during lovemaking, an opposite effect can often occur— unrelieved emotional tensions that will keep you awake after lovemaking. This is especially prevalent with women, who frequently take longer to reach orgasm and often fail to reach release during intercourse. They then lie in bed highly charged with energy, while the man falls blissfully asleep. This is a more serious cause of regular insomnia than is usually admitted, and is only relieved through masturbation, through getting up and doing something to dispel the sexual frustration, or through discussing the problem with your lover so that resolution of a positive nature is found between the two of you. Otherwise, frustration equals sleeplessness.

Healthy Diet for Sleep

Often people have difficulty in falling asleep because of their regular eating habits in the evening. For instance, a diet heavy in meat, dairy, and other high-fat foods is hard to digest, and can cause complications in falling asleep. Overeating of any food will have the same effect.

But what has recently been proven as most problematical in causing poor sleep is eating too late in the evening. Your stomach and intestines function differently at night than they do in the daytime. Optimal conditions exist in the stomach for digesting food during rest-time after lunch. The worst conditions exist when you go to bed and to sleep for the night. These bad conditions are generated by a change in functioning of the large intestine, because during sleep the intestines do not actively perform the absorption process which they do so well during the daytime.

The biochemical result is this: fermentation actually starts to take place in the large intestine, and an alcohol-base condition is created. This alcohol passes into your bloodstream, according to experimental reports, and creates a somewhat poisoned condition in your body during your sleep. This is why you so often wake up feeling like you have a hangover after eating a late meal, even if you didn't drink any alcohol that evening. The alcohol poisoning which you experience through this process also causes bad dreams, so that your sleep is fitful instead of restful.

This new medical information should be taken seriously to heart if insomnia or fitful sleeping is a problem, especially if you find yourself waking up in the middle of the night feeling sick and in bad emotional condition. Certainly the psychological sources we discussed in earlier chapters can be principal factors in your fitful sleep, but your late-night eating habits might be greatly aggravating the condition as well.

So I recommend that you reestablish your eating rituals (for these are certainly primary rituals in our lives) so that you eat your heaviest meal at lunch. And then for dinner, eat early and light.

By the way, there is some truth to the old wives' tale that a glass of warm milk before bedtime helps you to sleep.

Milk contains a substance which is presently being studied by researchers because it in fact tends to induce drowsiness. So if you enjoy it, the ritual of a warm cup of milk at night might be helpful—but avoid chocolate, since it contains caffeine. Also, of course, if insomnia is any kind of problem to you, cut out *all* sources of caffeine from your diet— certainly after lunch, and if possible completely. Note that this includes Coke with caffeine, candy with chocolate, black and green teas, etc. For many people, even one cup of coffee in the morning will disturb sleep patterns that night. If insomnia is a problem, cut out all caffeine!

Having a sugary dessert after dinner will likewise cause sleeping problems, since the sugar will be an active ingredient in causing the alcohol fermentation in your intestines while you sleep.

What About the Nightcap Routine?

For hundreds of years doctors have been recommending that patients with sleeping problems take a nightcap before retiring, because a shot of alcohol seems to help induce sleep. Is this true?

It is certainly true that one small drink of sherry, or a single beer perhaps, does temporarily generate relaxation in the body. It can also help the mind to relax and let go of worries. So getting to sleep can sometimes be encouraged through a nightcap.

However, after a few hours, the effects of alcohol on the system tend to reverse themselves, causing fitful sleep for the second half of the night. With this in mind, it seems that the recommendation of alcohol as a sleep aid is not a good idea on a regular basis.

Furthermore, what has been found is that most people who begin with one drink before bedtime start to take more than one drink—and as the ritual drink becomes a ritual of several drinks before bed, the entire tragedy of alcohol dependence begins to develop.

Almost all alcoholics complain regularly of sleep problems. Much of what I told you earlier about sleeping pills applies equally to alcohol. As you become dependent on the drug, you have to take more and more on a nightly basis to achieve a sleep state. And whenever you try to cut down on your intake, you get hit with rebound insomnia, which is worse than your condition before you started using alcohol to put you to sleep.

The old wives' tale and doctors' recommendation of a drink before bedtime might sometimes be perfectly fine, especially if you have had an extremely stressful day and need a little help to unwind. But as a regular bedtime ritual, it is very dangerous. If you are drinking at night more than two or three times a week, you should realize that you have a drinking dependency and that something should be done about it before serious consequences develop. The positive suggestions I'm making in this chapter should offer you alternative rituals to nurture as you strive to put aside the questionable ritual of alcohol. And many community programs are available if you need further help.

A Proper Hour for Hitting the Sack

As children we were usually put to sleep quite early in the evening, at six, seven, or eight o'clock at the latest. Then as we grew older and needed less sleep, we started to go to bed at later and later hours. At what time did you go to bed when you were five? When you were fifteen? When you were twenty-one?

There is of course no set time of the evening when one should go to bed. Many of us have jobs which force us to sleep at all times of the night and day. The principle to hold in mind is this—never force yourself to get into bed before you are able to go to sleep. The proper time to go to bed is when you are sleepy.

It takes time, a week or two, to readjust your sleeping times if you find they are presently not optimum for a good night's sleep. For instance, you might be forcing yourself to go to bed an hour or two too early, based on old routines which no longer apply to your sleeping needs. Maybe you only need seven hours of sleep, for instance, but have always thought you should try to get eight. This forced concept of the "adequate" amount of sleep often causes pseudo-insomnia.

What is important is to make sure that you set a particular

waking time, and adhere to that specific time on a regular basis. Wake up the same time each day as a beginning point, and then let your nighttime habits arrange themselves comfortably around that fixed time in the morning. If you fail to get up at the same time each morning, you will have serious difficulties in setting up a successful bedtime routine.

It is equally vital that you watch your habits at night to make sure you are not chronically pushing yourself to stay awake longer than you should. Curiously, people who tend to need more sleep each night than they allow themselves often create insomnia by forced wakefulness long into the night. This usually comes about because such people actually thrive on eight or nine or (like Albert Einstein) ten or even twelve hours of sleep a night, but they were conditioned in early adulthood to believe that anything over eight hours is indulgence and not good for alertness and performance.

These people use coffee, problem-solving work, and social activities to artificially stimulate them beyond their natural bedtimes. The result is a basic violation of the sleep cycles, which would naturally start an hour or two, or even three, before they actually are going to bed—and as you now know quite well, this means a loss of vital delta sleep each night.

So see what happens to you if you reduce artificial stimulations during the evening, certainly after ten o'clock. Give yourself a chance to relax into the evening, and begin to discover when you naturally begin to move toward the sleep state. I can't overemphasize the need for this reflection upon and possible readjustment of your sleeping habits.

Sleep-Time Rituals

Let's look with a little more depth into exactly what you do during the half hour before you climb into bed. Hopefully you have begun to make your complete list already, and will continue with this reflective process for the next few days and nights.

What I want to explore with you at this point is the extent to which you have turned your nightly habits into helpful rituals. Key to this transformation is your becoming conscious and appreciative of your rituals. For instance, when you are sitting in your favorite chair watching television (not so good) or reading or talking (much better), there comes a certain moment when the idea of bedtime comes into your mind, right?

This is the beginning of your bedtime ritual sequence, and becoming more conscious of when you feel this inner urge to begin a movement toward your bed and sleep is a vital step in learning how to use this half hour as meaningful preparation for sleep.

Sleep is something which must be surrendered to, in order for it to come and take you off into slumberland. If your mind is in tense problem-solving activity around bedtime, such surrender is directly thwarted, as we have seen. You need to learn how to shift your attention directly to the rituals you are going to perform in the last half hour before getting into bed if you want powerful help in breaking free of the mind-states which are the prime culprits of insomnia.

And this shifting of your attention to the physical rituals you are going to perform is one of the best ways to induce sleep that I have found.

Please understand that I am now leading you into the development of a routine which takes time to master. Don't think I am expecting you to perfect your mental shifting in a couple of nights. Give yourself a couple of weeks to explore what I mean by mental shifting and the power of nighttime rituals.

Again: you feel the beginning of the desire to go to bed, and then you act. You get up at some point and head in the general direction of your bedroom. This is a muscular event—and what you want to do at this point is to turn your attention to how you feel in your body. What is your breathing like just before you get up to go to bed? Are you feeling tense or relaxed? And do you really feel ready for sleep, or are you just pushing yourself because it is a certain time?

If it is "time to go to bed" by the clock, but if you don't feel tired yet, then *please* don't activate your bedtime rituals just yet! Instead, do this: get up and do some movements which will release the final tensions in your body, so that the urge to relax in bed and go to sleep can come to you naturally. Very often, if you just lie down on the floor and do very simple leg lifts, knee rolls, yoga stretches, etc., you will quickly discover that you are feeling too tired to continue with the exercises—and this is when you feel the readiness for bed!

Many clients I have worked with in this regard find that they quickly turn evening exercises into that first ritual which leads to a good night's sleep. At a certain time they discipline themselves to put the book down, turn off the damned television (forgive me my prejudice), say good night to their friends, and lie down on their backs to do their bedtime exercises. Such beginning discipline is necessary in most cases to overcome your inertia, lethargy, depression perhaps, and shift from inaction into action. It is a magical thing to do, this lying down on your back NOT in bed at first, but in another room on the floor. Tensions let go quickly, and if you do exercises until the urge to stop and go to bed comes over you, you can be almost sure that you have relieved yourself of most of the physical causes of insomnia, while shifting your consciousness away from the psychological habits that plague poor sleepers.

The trick of all this, of course, is in the shifting of your attention from thoughts to sensations, from past-future mental fixations to the present moment of your body and its constantly changing inputs of inner muscular sensations, sensory experience, and the emotional sense of well-being which comes from stretching movements. If you need to, also breathe through the mouth and discharge emotions vocally.

And then when the urge for bed comes genuinely over you, it is time to make another major move—surrendering to your desire and heading for your bed!

Rather than automatically walking to your bedroom, it is crucial to first acknowledge your body's desire for sleep; to say, "Okay, great idea, I agree with you, it's time to go to bed and have a good night's sleep." You should let yourself express your desire for sleep physically and vocally at this point, through a good stretch, several good yawns, and the accompanying sounds of pleasure and satisfaction.

Then you get up from your chair, or from the floor if you did some exercises, and act out your desire. Notice that you are doing something each night that is a fulfillment of your desires. You are doing something very nice for yourself. See this; acknowledge it consciously. You are being friendly with yourself, and this act of friendship just before going to bed can make all the difference in whether you feel well-loved and ready for sleep.

This is especially important if you live alone and don't have anyone to say good night to. The ritual of saying good night is one of the keys to a good night's sleep because sleeping is basically a communal event. If you are living alone, you *must* make your *own* presence the essential relationship that helps you to fall asleep.

Saying "Good Night"

Watch how you turn out the lights in the living room. Do you do this automatically with no conscious meaning—or do you say good night to the room as you put it to sleep?

I find it very important that insomniacs find someone or something to say good night to every night. It doesn't seem to matter if you say good night to a dozen kids in the nursery or to the room you have been sitting in alone for the evening. What is crucial is the ritual, the conscious act of saying good night—because this ritual stimulates associations with past experiences of family living, and thus paves the way for a restful sleep. To summon up past memories and feelings of security and love—this is the principal purpose of nighttime rituals. You are tapping into a vast storehouse of positive associations with this good-night ritual. Perhaps it is quite natural for people to live more and more alone as they grow older. This is the nature of life in many respects. But it is also natural for older people to have many memories to live with, to be nurtured by, so that they can readily feel the presence of relationships even long gone on the physical plane—and by awakening these relationships through simple ritual associations, a sense of well-being and security can instantly be regained.

Of course if you live with people and are not the last to go to bed, you use the ritual of saying good night verbally, and physically perhaps, to wake up the feeling of communal well-being. A hug at night, or a kiss, when done in a conscious manner as a surrender ritual to retreat and sleep, can work wonders for breaking the insomnia curse.

Bathroom Routines

One way or the other, you leave your living spaces, say good night to this world, and retreat to your bathroom rituals. Again, the helping key is to do these rituals consciously, rather than thinking of other things while you do them. Brushing your teeth should be an enjoyable routine, or combing your hair, or taking care of your dentures. To enjoy this period of the evening is what you want to aim for—and it is easy if you just watch your breathing, notice your whole body standing there doing each step of the ritual, and open yourself to the magnetic pull of bed.

Sleep comes through so many small steps, one after another, each made consciously and with the anticipation of the release of finally lying down and surrendering to relaxation and mental freedom from the day's thoughts. If you don't do these steps consciously, don't tap into their hypnotic, progressive magic, then you will find yourself getting into bed wide awake, not prepared at all for sleep.

If you are preparing for bed with another person, it is important to give each other space for these rituals. Going to bed needs to be essentially a solitary meditation, because as soon as you start to drift into sleep, you are in fact moving into a solitary experience. So make sure that you don't socialize while doing your bedtime rituals, or again, you will get into bed still buzzing, not relaxed and prepared for sleep.

Most important, don't hurry a ritual. I remember a minister at my family church when I was young. He was somewhat manic, this guy, and he hurried through the entire service. Everything was in a rush somehow, and the result was that everyone felt unsatisfied afterward. When finally he was replaced by another minister, I recall the unexpected powerful impact of the service as it was performed slowly, with reverence and enjoyment of each moment in time.

It is with this sense of peace, of relaxed pleasure in the eternal *now*, that I recommend you do your half hour of preparations for bed. This should be the most beautiful time of the day, when you have finished everything and are finally free. Enjoy the moments. Feel the delicious pull of bed and sleep. And then head into the bedroom in a state of peace and eagerness for the ultimate surrender.

Tonight, observe yourself as you go through your bedtime routines, without trying to change anything at all. Simply see clearly how you perform the rituals of bedtime. Then tomorrow sit down and write in your sleep journal what you did the night before. Compare your routine with the one I discussed in this chapter. And reflect on how you might want to expand your bedtime routine in directions which would enhance its ritual aspects.

Right now, take a few minutes to see what is coming to mind about your general relationship with that vital half hour before you have your head on your pillow. Pause from reading, watch your breathing a bit, tune into the feelings in your heart, in your pelvis, in your whole body. And let your intuitive voice speak to you about your sleep habits.

CHAPTER ELEVEN

Fantasies that Induce Sleep

You have now said good night to the living room, to the bathroom, and are in your bedroom ready to finally hit the hay. Probably at this point you finish your preparations regarding what you will wear to bed. Different people prefer different degrees of dress and undress for bed. A general recommendation is that you sleep with as little encumbrance as possible. One specific change that has often helped clients is this: make one alteration in your sleeping clothes, to bring a sense of newness to your bedtime feelings if you have had a long bout with troubled sleep. Especially, see how you feel if you stop wearing anything below the waist. I mention this because people often carry with them old inhibitions and anxieties related to nakedness. To break free of this, to let yourself feel directly the luxuriance of skin against sheets can bring a sense of pleasure to that first minute of relaxation as you slide under the covers.

It is unfortunate that so many of us as little children had negative treatment related to our sleeping situations. Too many parents used sleeping habits as opportunities for applying moralistic lessons, for instance. And much anxiety, guilt, and shame has been associated with the very act of getting undressed, getting into nightclothes chosen by the parents, and getting into bed. Many children had to sleep with older brothers and sisters in the same bed, which in some cases created sexual embarrassment and trauma as puberty arrived.

Let's take a reading break right here so that you can pause, put the book aside, and open yourself to memories that rise effortlessly into your mind regarding how you felt getting into the various beds you have slept in. Breathe a few easy breaths, and remember each bed you slept in while you were growing up.

Once in bed, consider the blankets or comforters you sleep under. Are these comfy enough to stimulate associations with early-childhood blankets, or are you presently sleeping under unsatisfying covers? Furthermore, is your bed adequate for a comfortable night's sleep, or are you trying to make do with an overly soft, overly small, or overly hard bed?

Sometimes I recommend to clients with sleep disturbances that they get their very own comforter to sleep under, one which is theirs alone—rather than sharing space under sheets. The Europeans with their down comforters have perhaps the ideal sleeping concept, one which the American tradition has somehow lost. A comforter provides an exceptionally cozy womblike experience which sheets and blankets simply do not offer. If you want to enhance your sleeping situation, I recommend that you try a comforter, although this is of course an added expense, and not essential to the program.

We should also talk about the wisdom of sleeping alone, at least sometimes, even if you are living with your loved one. Sometimes two people in the same bed, no matter how much they love each other, disturb each other's sleep. Quite a number of times I have worked with clients with sleep complaints, only to find that when they simply started sleeping in separate beds, the sleep disorders disappeared completely. I am certainly not recommending this pattern for all couples. Many people absolutely love sleeping in the same bed with their living partner.

However, do look seriously into which pattern is best for you: sleeping under the same blankets in constant intimate contact throughout the night; sleeping in the same large bed with individual comforters for each of you to curl up under in somewhat separate space; or sleeping in different beds either in the same room or in separate rooms.

This can be a very touchy topic to bring up with your

mate, of course. Perhaps you need more of your own separate space in order to have a good night's sleep, but your mate needs your physical presence in order to sleep well. By considering the four possibilities listed in the previous paragraph, though, you should be able to reach a compromise that satisfies both of you.

What must be remembered concerning sleeping habits is that most of us grew up sleeping in our own separate beds, and often in our own bedrooms. Our basic childhood sleeping patterns were established in such solitary ways. But then suddenly we grew up and fell in love and bam! There went all our nocturnal peace and sense of separate space, violated by the loving presence of our sexual partner.

Many people simply cannot have a deep dream experience when they are sleeping with someone in the same bed. The very presence of another being so close beside them disturbs the peace they need in order to relax into a deep dream state, not to mention into delta sleep. When you consider the fact that this other person is liable to be having wild energetic dreams right when you are wanting to slip into deep sleep, the conflicts of sleeping with another person can be seen quite clearly.

The result is often that neither of the partners ever gets a really good night's sleep, year after year, throughout the relationship. They get enough good sleep to get by the next day, but there is a subtle loss which is experienced both in terms of dreams and delta sleep. I think for almost everyone there is a tradeoff between the wonderful deep sleep you have when sleeping alone in your own little world at night and the wonderful experience of having a loving warm body sleeping with you.

I have several times been accused of threatening to disrupt the basic foundation of marriage with my suggestions to consider sleeping separately. But there remains the reality to be dealt with—the presence of another sleeping person in bed with you while you are trying to have a good night's sleep can create a disturbance which negatively affects your sleep potential. You must consider this disturbance in contrast with the pleasures and security you gain through sleeping with your lover, and then decide which is most important to you at this point in your life.

If your sleep is not good in general, you should consider sleeping in a separate bed for at least a while, to see if this eases your insomnia. The best way to look at it is this: you can have all the pleasure of jumping into the same bed with your lover when there is a mutual desire for lovemaking. You can also certainly sleep together whenever you both want to. But perhaps you can reserve the freedom of sleeping in your own bed when you want to. This is optimum freedom in the sleeping situation. You can also join each other in the same bed upon waking, to share that beautiful beginning of the day skin to skin as much as you so desire.

I am emphasizing this sleeping-partner situation at great length because I suspect it is such a common problem among couples, going unrecognized for year after year. Most people would consider it somehow a threat to their relationship if their partner were to suddenly say, "Hey, honey, I think I want to sleep alone in a separate bed, is that okay with you?"

The reaction of the surprised partner is almost certainly "No! That's not okay with me. What do you mean, don't you love me anymore?"

I hope that this discussion can shed some dispassionate light on such a universal situation. The truth is that many relationships finally fall apart because of the partners living just one step too close to each other. Again we come to the question of dependency versus independence in relationships. Couples come together through the desire to overcome loneliness and a sense of separation. This is all good and fine. But often two people cement themselves into habits of relating which are so tight as to be suffocating. Still, out of fear of being alone again, neither of the partners dares risk saying, "I love you very deeply, but I also need my own solitary space sometimes in order to really be happy. Can I back away just a couple of steps so that I have a little breathing room? Like for instance, do you suppose I could start sleeping down the hall in the guest room when I want to, so that I can get a really good night's sleep when I need it?"

I can't go into this theme too deeply in the context of this book, but I hope that I have said enough to stimulate your reflection on this topic, and action if needed. If you really do love your partner, you aren't going to lose him or her if you act in this manner, I am almost certain. If your relationship is shaky already and your need for some solitary sleeping space is the straw that breaks the conjugal camel's back, then what can I say? Good luck in establishing realistic sleeping conditions in your next relationship. But my experience has shown that many more relationships have been saved by facing the conjugal bed dilemma honestly than have been damaged.

Of course for many of you, who are going to bed alone every night and wishing to high heaven that you had a good loving relationship and a partner to cuddle up with all night, this last discussion might have seemed extremely indulgent. Many more people suffer from insomnia because their bed is empty of a loving partner than because their bed is full of too much loving partner.

If you are alone and want to find someone to share your sleep with, your whole life with, then this is a situation requiring a special program in itself, which I have explored in my book *Finding Each Other*. Rather than trying to give here any summary of the process of searching for the person you need to satisfy your intimate needs, I should point you in the direction of that complete discussion.

However, regardless of what your intimate standing is right now, the question remains—how do you get to sleep tonight, while you are also working to resolve your long-term interpersonal needs?

You are in bed. You have gone through the preparation rituals faithfully, and yet when your head hits the proverbial pillow, you find yourself terribly awake, with no hope of sleep in sight. What can you do right at that point to help induce sleep?

In-Bed Procedures

First of all, go through the procedure I taught you earlier, of snuggling up under your covers and seeing if you can let go of present tensions and return to those good early-childhood feelings you used to have in bed. Use this regression technique to shift your consciousness effortlessly into the sleep mode. Every night practice this, even when sleep is easy, so that you develop a good solid relationship with the feeling of infantile bliss.

Secondly, if sleep does not come easily, roll onto your back and go through the mental relaxation meditation. Watch your breathing as every new breath comes without effort. . . . Expand your awareness to include your jaw muscles, and relax them with every new breath as well. . . . Then expand your awareness to include your pelvic region, and let this area move gently with every breath. . . . Focus on your toes and fingers in this relaxation process, moving them and encouraging relaxation throughout. . . . Once you have fully encountered your entire body lying here in the present moment, let yourself stretch and yawn a few delicious times, making good sighing sounds of pleasure as you tune deeper and deeper into the feeling of your body lying on the bed, relaxing step by step. . . . and now count your breaths as you move deeper into sleep.

If you relax into this meditation but still find that you are somehow agitated inside, with a mind that just doesn't feel ready to let go of its activities, you will do best to turn your mind's energies in the direction of some fantasy adventures.

Bedtime Fantasies

Human beings are both blessed and cursed with the ability to fantasize. As I mentioned earlier, worrying and chronic problem-solving are examples of fantasy activity which are prime causes of insomnia. But fantasies can also be put to very effective service in just the opposite direction—in stimulating feelings which lead to sleep.

Along with basic worries about survival, isolation, and hopelessness, as mentioned earlier, people also often lie in bed unable to sleep at night because of another important psychological condition—the feeling of somehow being inadequate, of lacking in the basic qualities which are needed in order to get out into the world and succeed in love and survival games.

Such a condition of a weak self-image so often accompanies the condition of insomnia that I want to dedicate the final part of this chapter to techniques for overcoming this feeling. As I suggested earlier, you can act during the daytime by giving yourself credit for whatever small or large achievements you might make. But at night, instead of lying there going over all the mistakes you have made, or fantasizing about terrible things that might befall you in the future because of your perceived inadequacies, you can reverse this habit and start imagining yourself in a new light.

Almost all children lie in bed imagining a wild assortment of fantasies in which they are the central character, and they are the champion! And it is this ability to see yourself in a positive light which we are going to turn to your advantage, in creating an emotional condition in the present moment which will induce sleep.

You simply lie there in bed, let your eyes close, notice your breathing a moment, and then see what comes to mind when you imagine that you are in a situation where you are doing something carefully, masterfully, and gracefully. It can be anything at all, either something you did actually in the past, or a fantasy of doing something in the future—or just a pure wild fantasy of any sort. Perhaps you are driving a car with perfect timing and control along a winding road; perhaps you are sanding a piece of wood until it is perfectly smooth to the touch; or you are playing an instrument with an orchestra, performing the solo lead in a concerto; or you are massaging your lover's body with strong loving strokes of your hands; or you are speaking in front of an audience that is listening eagerly to your every word; or you are making love with wild abandon, much to your partner's pleasure; or you are sitting quietly on a mountaintop, meditating on the universe, your whole being radiating in eternal bliss . . .

See what comes to mind now as you put the book aside, close your eyes, and open yourself to any fantasy in which you are doing something with great mastery, finesse, and pleasure.

Beyond Bad Dreams

Many people suffering from insomnia are caught up in a condition which I haven't mentioned until now, but which must come before we end our discussion. We have spoken only a little about dreams as related to sleeplessness. But in fact many people lie in bed at night unable to get to sleep, specifically because they are afraid of terrible dreams that might come, dreams similar to ones which have scared them before, and which they dread experiencing again.

Little children naturally go through phases of having bad dreams as they struggle to come to conscious grips with one difficult reality after another in life. Many children regularly have nightmares, filling them with terror and apprehension related to sleep in general. But usually these apprehensions are overcome as the various causes of the nightmares are worked through in everyday life.

For adults, however, the fear of nightmares can return to plague the dark hours of each day. People seem to awaken from terrible dreams when the dreams start to hit too closely to one's darkest desires. People who are blocking angry feelings toward an employer, for instance, often have violent dreams which are trying to release the anger through fantasy. This is at least the psychoanalytical understanding of dreaming, and I think there is more than a grain of truth to it.

But if an inhibited person starts to dream of actually socking his employer right in the nose, then this dream becomes too threatening to the dreamer—and he wakes up from a terrible dream of violence. Usually the violence has been taken one step into fantasy, and the person might dream of cutting off his employer's head with a machete—or as is often the case, the dreamer will reverse the direction of the aggression and dream that someone is trying to cut his or her head off with a machete.

In any case, the dreamer wakes up from a terrible dream and dreads falling asleep and risking another such nightmare. The result is most certainly insomnia at its very worst. And what a terrible predicament it is, to need to sleep very badly, but to fear sleeping at the same time. I think all of us have known this condition at least a few times.

What can realistically be done when bad dreams and the fear of bad dreams are ruining your sleep night after night? Certainly various forms of therapy can be of significant help in directly working through the buried emotions and fantasies which are generating terrible nighttime dreams. If this is a serious problem for you, perhaps professional help might be worthwhile.

But you can also help yourself, especially by devoting regular time to the emotional release and balancing program I outlined earlier. Let me walk you a few steps deeper into the process, so you can have a clearer focus.

During daytime sessions, retreat for twenty minutes or so and lie down on your back. Loosen or take off your clothes so that you feel physically free. And simply start breathing freely through your mouth, with deep conscious inhales and exhales. Do this for several minutes. To add to the breathing exercise, charge your body by moving your arms and legs as if you are running, so your breathing deepens.

Then just relax, but continue breathing through your mouth even if this is at first difficult. Your habits will try to block your deep breathing, because you will almost certainly start to feel inhibited feelings and fantasies starting to emerge from inside you.

At this point, set your imagination free to come up with any images which might spring to mind, to accompany the emotions you are feeling. Especially open yourself to fantasies of aggression toward people in your present life or from past periods of your life. Imagine all the terrible, monstrous things which you usually keep yourself from even thinking for a moment. Let yourself kill your boss, smash your momma to bits, drive a cement truck over your father, throw your kids in a bottomless pit—give vent to all those infantile emotions which are a part of everyone's psyche but which you have perhaps repressed and thus turned into monsters inside you.

Also imagine all the most terrible things that could happen to yourself, especially all the horrible ways you might be killed. Keep on playing out these fantasies for several sessions of daytime self-therapy, until you have released them into the light and put them in their proper place, which is as a tiny fantasy part of your emotional being. This infantile dimension of your psyche will always be part of you; there is no getting away from it, as you have found out the hard way through your disturbed sleep. The only positive step is to admit to the fantasies, experience them in daytime sessions, and discharge the emotional pressure you have been generating to block their expression.

As you experience your repressed fantasies, you will also begin to make contact with the actual real-life situations in which you need to be more assertive, where what you need is not to cut off your boss's head with a machete, but to stand up to him or her and speak your mind clearly and powerfully. It might take you months to arrive at this final breakthrough, but every step in the right direction will feel wonderful. Your anxieties will dissipate as you face your dangers and build up your sense of self-confidence.

Sleep disturbances, as we have seen, come both from your present life situations and also from past situations which are not fully resolved in your inner being. Both of these dimensions need to be looked into, if you are to progress into sleep-full nights. What you need to do is to act—to regularly do the various sessions I have taught you, so that you shift from being a victim to being in positive control of your life.

Then, when it is time to sleep at night, you can turn your conscious attention to the techniques you have learned for inducing relaxation, for quieting your thinking mind, and for acting out the rituals which lead to sleep.

CHAPTER TWELVE

Advanced Suggestions

I should point out that there are times when you do benefit from lying sleepless in bed thinking through a difficult problem. Part of life does involve struggling late into the night sometimes, in order to see to the center of a situation and decide how to act the next morning. If you are overly dictatorial with your mind, always trying to turn it off at 10:25 in the evening rather than going with unexpected wakeful flows now and then, you will create inner conflicts which certainly upset your sleep.

I want to make clear, however, the distinction between occasional sleepless nights and chronic insomnia which plagues you every night no matter what is going on in your daytime life. It is quite normal for everyone to have occasional difficulties in life which keep one awake at night. If you don't sleep much for one or two nights, your performance the next day is not going to be seriously upset, so don't worry about it. After an hour or so of problem-solving use the techniques I've been showing you, so that you do get enough sleep. But don't worry about a little lost sleep here and there.

And when something really traumatic does happen to you, such as the death of a friend, the loss of a job, or even the collapse of a long-cherished belief, don't be overly upset when you have several nights of sleep disturbances. Roll with the punches, use my suggestions to transcend your traumatic emotions—but keep in mind that the loss of friend or a valued job does create turbulence within you. And there is no easy way through grief. You have to experience suffering and emotional contraction in order to weather the storm through to the other end of the growth period. There is a certain therapeutic need for tossing and turning at night, as your soul wrestles with the situation and finally moves into acceptance and transcendence.

But when you seem to be unable to sleep over a longer period of time, and when your insomnia seems to be rooted in a more general free-floating anxiety and sense of aggression or depression, then along with using the sleep suggestions I have been offering you will also need to look more deeply into your long-term personality qualities which are instigating your sleepless nights.

I hope that for many of you these discussions will shed enough light for you to be able to work through your own problems. You will need to go back and reread this book a number of times, so that the words sink deeper and deeper into your mind. And you will also need to be brave enough to risk looking at parts of yourself which you usually avoid. The challenge is a big one, but one which most of you can in fact take on and be victorious with.

For those of you who feel that you definitely need some professional guidance, person-to-person, my advice is to seek out a very good therapist to help you get right to the source of your emotional blockages, helping you to consciously release your old fears and rages and become good friends with the very emotions which you are presently afraid of— and which are undermining your potential for deep restful sleep.

Although the direct cause of sleepless nights does seem to be buried emotional turmoil and pressures, it should be emphasized that it is your mind's thinking habits which are chronically stimulating the emotional turmoil. When you lie in bed, the instigator of tensions in the body is almost always thoughts in the mind. If no images and ideas come to a person's mind, and no environmental stress is perceived through the senses, then in fact one's emotions are quiet. Emotions are responses—this is important to remember.

Therefore, when you are seeking release from insomnia, don't look just to emotional release. Look also to your habits of thought. Any good therapist knows this and will help you along the path to freedom from compulsive worrying habits. But you can help yourself as well. Let me take you a step deeper into the process.

Quieting Compulsive Thoughts

I have shown you how to shift your attention from thinking into perceptual awareness of your body and the world around you in the present moment. This is certainly an effective means for quieting the thinking mind. When you also count your breaths to yourself, you activate the mind with busywork which also keeps thought-flows from happening, as we have already seen.

But sometimes even these semi-hypnotic techniques for inducing sleep can fail you, and you are left still caught up in the overwhelming tense activities of your unstoppable mind, and you feel there is no hope for you.

Right at this point, it is vital to let go of all the techniques I have taught you for trying to fall asleep. Accept that your mind is dominant for the moment. And instead of feeling depressed or angry at yourself, just do the following. Use a judo move on your mind! Accept its busy thinking-thinking-thinking without any resistance at all. Give it full permission to carry on with its compulsive behavior.

The trick you are going to play on your thinking mind is this: you are not going to identify completely with your thoughts. You are not going to be completely caught up with the meaning of what you are thinking about. You are instead going to practice a special meditation in which you step back a few steps from the constant flow of words going past your consciousness, so that you can observe yourself thinking.

Watching oneself in the process of thinking is one of the spiritual challenges of utmost importance for all of us. If only we can gain a little distance from the chronic flow of words which dominate our minds, we can see the repetitive nature of our thoughts and move beyond the unconscious mental habits which hold us in limited participation with the world around us.

Ultimately, your insomnia should be seen as a blessing in disguise. You are finally being forced, through the symptom of not being able to get to sleep, to step back and take a look at the way in which your mind has been programmed to function, and the way in which it is running out of control in your life. This is where I find the greatest value in consciously exploring insomnia with a client. Symptoms in one's body and behavior are always indicators of something deep down that needs to be dealt with, something which is throwing the entire system of the mind/body/spirit off-center.

And by having to consciously deal with your symptom of a chronically restless mind which generates an inability to sleep, by having to step back to see what is wrong, you gain the immense blessing of finally dealing with mental habits which are probably upsetting the entire realm of your life, not just your sleepless nights.

This entire book has been building toward this point, where we have an understanding of insomnia which enables us to see insomnia in perspective, in its symptomatic role of getting our attention so that we will begin to consciously deal with old habits which are driving us to ruin.

All through our discussion, you have seen how your thoughts, and more specifically your habits of thinking about certain topics over and over and over again, serve to stimulate chronic emotional contractions, which in turn generate chronic muscular tensions, which then keep you from relaxing at night and drifting into much-needed sleep.

I have shown you ways for quieting the mind which usually work. But when nothing works, you have no choice but to confront your mind itself, to separate yourself from your flow of thoughts so that you can see that you are more than thoughts, that your consciousness is much greater than just the cognitive flow of words through your mind.

But how in a pragmatic way can we make this great step into gaining a perspective on the chronic flow of thoughts through our minds?

I am going to say this very simply. You are in bed or sitting up late at night, unable to sleep. Your mind is tense with thoughts and images, your body is tense with emotional knots. You can't do relaxation meditations because you are too nervous, agitated, or depressed.

So simply do this. Let your thoughts continue to flow, and at the same time, be aware of your breathing. Expand your awareness so that you are with your thoughts, but you are also with your breathing, both happening at the same time, and both being watched by your consciousness.

This primal trick of meditation, this expanding of one's awareness to include two happenings at once, is at the core of breaking free of compulsive behavior of any kind. You have already exercised your ability to do this, in the relaxation meditation in which you observe the sensation of air flowing through your nose, and at the same time observe the sensation of movement in your body as you breathe. That meditation is perfect preparation for doing this more advanced meditation of watching your thoughts as they go by, while also watching the air flowing in and out your nose, and the movement of your body as you breathe.

We have simply expanded the two-part meditation into a three-part meditation. Please note that making the additional step is just as effortless as making the first two steps. The expansion of awareness is not an effortful act. You cannot force yourself to be more aware. You can only relax your awareness, in order to let it expand. This is one of the ultimate principles of life, and it applies directly to the relaxation which needs to happen inside you if you are to let go of thoughts and fall asleep. Falling asleep happens to require an expansion of consciousness in which you tune into your whole body (what a great expansion!) and let your spirit move beyond your conceptual world into that vast realm of consciousness which includes dreaming, and which also includes the stage-four delta sleep state in which you are in fact expanded infinitely in all directions—thus the power of phase-four sleep to induce a recharging of your batteries.

Relaxation leads to sleep. The expansion of consciousness leads to relaxation. So the path to sleep is simple. You have only to learn how to relax your mind. And the beauty of the meditation I am presently teaching you is that by some miracle no psychologist has yet to explain, when you become aware of your breathing while you watch your thoughts going by, when you gain an expanded perspective of your habitual thoughts which run through your mind over and over again—when you stop identifying with these thoughts and reacting to them emotionally, you begin to relax!

This happens as a natural process. Your breathing will

begin to relax first, as it always does when you take time to observe it in the present moment. Then your whole body will start to relax. And then your thoughts begin to become quiet. It is a process the great spiritual masters have known for countless generations. Jesus taught this peace of mind as a primary pillar of his message. He preached peace. What I have explained to you here is simply a logical account of how peace is attained, in its purest form.

Even though Jesus was primarily a man of peace, he was also a very clear and great thinker. There is nothing wrong with thinking—what is problematic is when your thinking machine becomes a loop tape, playing back the same old worries and anxieties over and over again in infinite variety but always with the same theme.

Compulsive thinking is exactly this—repetitive thought patterns which you cannot turn off, which stimulate negative emotional contractions in your body and dominate consciousness with all their shouting and worrying. And the only way to break free of this pattern is to step back and see that it is in fact happening.

You now know the process for stepping back, the judo move which can transform your life—while your mind is busy thinking, expand your awareness so that you are also watching the sensations coming into your mind from your breathing, one breath after the other. By pulling your awareness back in this fashion, you then actually observe yourself thinking. It is a most amazing experience. I wish to God that we would teach our children how to do this early in life, so that we would all grow up with clearer, less compulsive thoughts.

Hopefully, as human beings we are evolving in this direction of being less compulsive, of having some distance from our own thoughts, so that we can act in more peaceful, clearheaded ways.

So the path away from insomnia is a path into a new realm of consciousness. By being provoked into doing something about your insomnia, you have found yourself evolving into a more expansive experience both of yourself and of the world around you. Your insomnia ultimately is a blessing in disguise, and I hope that I have given you the practical psychological and spiritual tools for meeting the challenge of your sleepless nights, and turning the challenge into a beautiful movement forward in your life.

As a daily meditation, a few times each day for a few minutes learn to watch your thoughts going by. Become adept at this simple expansion of consciousness, so that when you really need to do it well, when you are unable to sleep because your old compulsive thinking habits have you in their grip, you will be prepared to do this meditation under stress, and succeed with it!

Right now, as our last meditation break in the book, why don't you take a few moments to put the book aside, and begin to be aware of your breathing and the flow of words through your mind, at the same time.

Final Words

You now have a complete set of exercises and meditations to put to use to help you overcome your problems in getting a good night's sleep. There are twenty-five different suggestions you can now turn to at any time, for guidance along the path that leads away from insomnia.

The question remaining resides squarely in your side of the court—to what extent are you ready to act on your own behalf, to consciously evolve into a new relationship with yourself, with your nighttime self in particular, so that you can break the curse of sleepless nights and start enjoying restful nights again?

At the same time that I want to encourage you to push ahead through the various programs into the realms of a good night's sleep, I also want to caution you against pushing too hard too fast. Growth of our inner selves is a delicate process that does take time. Insomnia habits are often quite ingrained into our minds and bodies, and they cannot be simply dynamited out of the way. They must be seen clearly, accepted in the present moment, and then step by step gently transformed into more satisfying patterns of nighttime behavior.

There are three different times in each day when you can pick up this book and choose a particular reflection or meditation to do, to encourage a good night's sleep. During the daytime hours, it is extremely worthwhile to set aside at least one five-to-ten minute period when you pause to focus your full attention on this vital question of restful sleep. Choose a meditation from the twenty-five listed in the front of the book, read the related material, and then do the actual meditation. If you can develop the discipline of turning your attention each day to at least one of the outlined exercises, you will accelerate your progression out of insomnia. I hope you take on this challenge of developing enough discipline to do a meditation a day, during the day. Not only your sleep life but the entire quality of your conscious experience of life will be enhanced by such a reflective discipline on a daily basis.

A second time to develop such a discipline is in the evening, when instead of watching the boob tube or doing some other activity, you give yourself at least ten or fifteen minutes to sit down with this book, read a chapter, and do the meditations suggested for that chapter. In this way, every two weeks or so you will cover the entire scope of the programs. And it is the entire scope of the book taken as a whole which affords you optimum success with the programs. The effort to do this nightly reading and meditation will certainly pay high rewards, as you develop a beautiful habit of regularly pausing to look inward, to tune into your breathing and whole body here in the present moment, and in this expanded sense of your presence to reflect on different qualities of the sleep experience.

Even once you have conquered insomnia and are sleeping like a baby again, I highly recommend that you continue such a reflection process on a daily basis, so that you stay in tune with your inner feelings, and through such preventative awareness make sure that you don't slip into the hell of chronic insomnia ever again. All of us face this challenge of remaining in harmony with our feelings and thoughts so that our sleep is relatively untouched by daytime traumas.

The third time when you will want to reach for this book is when you are in the middle of a bout of insomnia and want some "first-aid" help in getting to sleep at night. You can either read through whole chapters which seem to speak most deeply to your present feelings and upset, or you can look at the list of twenty-five meditations, and let your eyes just rest on the list while you watch your breathing—until your eyes almost magically come to rest on the particular meditation that would be best to do at the moment. This bit of "magic" in selecting the proper meditation almost always works to guide you perfectly where you need to turn your attention, since it allows your intuitive mind to do the selecting.

Many of the meditations, reflections, and exercises on the list require that you read the suggestion, then put the book aside and try to guide yourself through the suggestion. For some of you, and certainly all of you some of the time, such self-guidance by reading and then doing will work beautifully. At times, however, you might want further help in moving deeply into the experiences being suggested by the exercise. If so, let me list alternative techniques for gaining guidance from an external source.

First of all, you can tape-record some of the most important exercises, using a microphone and tape recorder and reading or paraphrasing the suggestions from the book. This is very helpful for many people, especially in the middle of the night when it can be of great help to just flip a switch, relax in bed, and listen to a voice gently guiding you through the programs that lead to sleep.

If you find it hard to follow your own voice, perhaps you can ask a friend to record the various parts of the book which you want to delve deeply into. Often the sound of someone else's voice works better as a guide than your own, but this is purely individual.

For years now, I have been making my own tapes in this manner, for clients to take home and use during the week between sessions. Such auditory support in one's own home environment can be extremely helpful in generating rapid personal growth on many fronts of life. And in fact, many guided sessions which I use regularly in my practice translate perfectly onto guided cassette sessions which can be taken home and listened to many many times, especially when the suggestions are open-ended, so that each time you listen to a suggestion you go deeper into the experience, and explore the expansive realms of consciousness each suggestion opens up to you.

Although I tend to lose money in the process of producing such cassette programs, I do consider them invaluable aids to a book such as this, for those of you who would appreciate a friendly voice to lead you effortlessly into the various exercises and meditations we have been learning for inducing sleep. So you will find at the end of the book a list of available cassette programs which will augment your progress in attaining a good night's sleep on a regular basis. They are not essential to success, but certainly in many cases quite helpful.

And of course if you find that you are having serious difficulties, even with cassette assistance, in getting to the heart of your sleep problem, there will perhaps come a time when you want to seek out professional help in this regard.

But for most of you, the programs in this book should give you the practical tools for helping yourself into better sleep experiences in the near future. I wish you best of luck, and hope that this book serves as a manual the rest of your life, in keeping your sleep life in optimum shape!

Supporting Cassette Programs

There are two different times in your evening routine when the help of a guiding voice can prove invaluable to you, as you move toward sleep. First of all, it is helpful to be able to put a relaxing cassette on just before you go to bed, so that you are effortlessly moved into a state of mind and body which leads naturally into a satisfying sleep. Secondly, there are the more difficult times when you simply cannot fall asleep, or wake up in the middle of the night and are unable to get back to sleep. In this second case, sometimes you need guidance in working through emotional tensions, resolving past experiences, and breaking free of physical contractions which thwart sleep.

There are five cassette tapes, each with two programs aimed at the various needs of those of you who suffer from sleepless nights. The first two tapes are guided sessions to use before going to bed, or when you wake up and need a simple program to help you drift back to sleep. The third and fourth tapes are specific sessions for helping you to work through the problems we have been exploring in the book. And the fifth tape, a music tape without a guiding voice, is for anytime you want to relax and ease into a more comfortable, enjoyable state of mind and body.

Sleep Cassette One: A Good Night's Sleep

Side A: "Welcome To A Good Night's Sleep" is a combination of special music composed to induce relaxation and sleep, and a gentle voice which guides your attention calmly through the various relaxation techniques you have learned in the book. This basic sleep-induction program will help ease you quickly into a deep satisfying sleep.

Side B: "Roundtrip Ticket To Dreamland" is a continuation of this sleep-induction program, so that you can go deeper into the relaxation process if you need more time and guidance before falling asleep. The music in itself should smooth out your tensions effortlessly, while the guiding voice calms your mind, relaxes your tense muscles, and leads you off into dreamland.

Sleep Cassette Two: Inner Peace in Action

Side A: "Everyday Peace" is a special program which complements the sleep programs, offering soothing music and a guiding voice which leads you into a pure calm experiencing of the present moment. The expansion of your awareness beyond thoughtflows, and into a quiet enjoyment of your perceptual realms of consciousness, prepares you to drift into sleep at night, and to enjoy a relaxing break during the day.

Side B: "Serene Contemplations" features very soft bells and chimes which sound like distant church bells and a guiding voice that leads you away from emotional tensions, and into a quiet contemplative state of mind. Again, you can listen to this program during the day for regaining peace of mind, and also use the tape as a complement to the sleep programs, to gently induce the state of peace which comes just before you drop off to sleep.

Sleep Cassette Three: Memory and Fantasy Adventures

Side A: "Memory Excursions" begins with a relaxing few moments while you bring yourself fully into the present moment. Then off you go into a dozen different realms of your past, where you remember all the different positive experiences of your childhood, so that you make contact with your youthful spirit and break free of your adult worries and tensions. Often it is both therapeutic and a great pleasure to remember yourself enjoying life as a child, so that you bring this simple spirit into the present moment again. And each time you listen to the open-ended suggestions, you will find yourself going into new realms of memory, as your past expands into a full universe to explore and relax into.

Side B: "Free Fantasy Adventures" takes you off into a perfect guided fantasy vacation through a calm beautiful country world where everything is harmonious, and you walk, swim, lay in the sun, hike over a hill, watch the sun set, and then return to your ideal fantasy home where your friends await you for dinner, music, relaxation . . . and then it is time for bed, you take a good hot bath, then slip under the sheets and drift into dreamland. . . . This guided-fantasy technique for moving into sleep is one of the most powerful ones we have found to date, and should serve you very well. Again, you can listen to this tape a thousand times, and go deeper and deeper into the guided imagery, as you become more familiar with the world you learn to explore in your imagination. And the ending of the perfect day is of course the beginning of a good night's sleep!

Sleep Cassette Four: Emotional Release and Balancing

Side A: "Emotional Balancing" guides you through a basic therapy process for feeling each of the twelve primary emotions for a short time, then letting go and moving into the next emotion, and then the next . . . so that by the end of the session, you have experienced and consciously released a spectrum of emotions through the guidance of the speaking voice. This is a very powerful technique for resolving your emotional conflicts, one I use regularly in my therapy work, and which adapts itself beautifully to a cassette program you can use regularly at home. This program should prove itself especially helpful when you are awake at night, tense with emotional conflicts, and unable to let go of them. Just put on the tape and go through the balancing process, and you will usually be ready for sleep afterwards.

Side B: "Emotional Release and Healing" provides you with additional guidance you will sometimes need, when you go through the emotional balancing process and are still charged with one or two particular emotions. This session brings you through a professional emotional release experience, encouraging you to express your pent-up feelings, and then guiding you through a successful resolution of these feelings, and focusing on a relaxing, emotional healing period to end the session in a calm, reflective, relaxed state, ready for sleep.

Sleep Cassette Five: Zen Tunes for Relaxation

For years now I have been exploring the use of music as a vehicle for relaxation, contemplation, and the encouragement of peace of mind. For several years while I was working in Europe, I was lucky enough to explore a new form of music with a group of excellent professional jazz and classical musicians. The final result was *"Zen Tunes,"* an integrated flow of twenty-four short spontaneous compositions which guide you through many different meditative states. The music is relaxing without being repetitive, peaceful while also musically interesting. The instruments are natural ones, piano, guitar, both silver and wooden flutes, soft bells, fretless bass, slide guitars, harmonic voices . . . This is music you can listen to any time of day when you want a calming influence, and of course when you want to drift off to sleep.

If you would like information on any of these supporting programs, you can write to Maurizia Zanin, John Selby Programs, PO Box 8320, Santa Fe, NM 87504. Information on professional sleep-disturbance centers in your region is also available upon request.

WHEN BAD THINGS HAPPEN TO GOOD PEOPLE

HAROLD KUSHNER

Life-affirming views on how to cope with hard times and personal pain.

"Must reading for everyone who deals with tragedy."
Art Linkletter

"Provocative and comforting answers to the universal question: why me?" *Redbook*

"A book that all humanity needs."
Norman Vincent Peale

"Harold Kushner deals with the theme of inexplicable illness with deep insight and provides invaluable reassurance." Norman Cousins